Advance Praise for *Preemie Care*

"Lasby and Sherrow have produced an incredible resource—a go-to reference for families experiencing the birth of a preemie. The intimate vignettes from those who have walked this path will be of great comfort to preemie parents. I highly recommend this book to anyone who needs clarity on their journey through the NICU and support in the transition home."

DR. MICHAEL NARVEY

neonatologist and creator of *All Things Neonatal*

"Lasby and Sherrow share a vitally important perspective on all the challenges, big and small, that families encounter in the first few months after discharge. The authors have helped countless families face all the issues that arise and how to manage them practically. Filled with useful, understandable background information and invaluable tips, this phenomenal resource will benefit any parent getting ready to go home with their precious new family member."

DR. DEBORAH CLARK

neonatologist, associate clinical professor, University of Calgary

"Having a premature baby is a life-changing experience full of fear, stress, and uncertainty. Written by two highly experienced NICU nurses, *Preemie Care* provides a lifeline to guide parents through this challenging journey."

DEB FRASER

neonatal nurse practitioner and editor of

Neonatal Network: Journal of Neonatal Nursing

"In the NICU nurse's toolbox, this book will be an excellent resource to offer parents, providing them the opportunity to explore what they'll encounter during and after their NICU stay; describing the NICU environment and a typical preemie's medical journey; and giving practical tips for healthy coping. Fellow NICU colleagues will applaud them both for meeting this need and supporting our families."

DR. AMY WRIGHT

president, Canadian Association of Neonatal Nurses; assistant professor, Lawrence S. Bloomberg Faculty of Nursing, University of Toronto

"This is a very comprehensive, practical book filled with advice for all who care for NICU babies. With their wealth of training and unique experiences, Lasby and Sherrow have provided the most important information around the NICU stay and the time beyond the NICU doors. They present complex information in a straightforward and personable way. As an NICU physician for more than forty years, I have heard many families and colleagues ask questions that are clearly answered and explained in this book."

DR. REG SAUVE

physician and professor emeritus, University of Calgary

"This book is just what parents have been waiting for to support their transition home from the NICU. It provides answers to questions that many parents may not think to ask themselves. I highly recommend *Preemie Care* to all NICU parents."

DEB MCNEIL

former NICU staff nurse, educator, clinical nurse specialist and manager, and current maternal child health scientist and professor, University of Calgary

"As a neonatal nurse practitioner, I help coordinate very complicated discharges as these very fragile babies go home with their families for the first time. Despite weeks of preparation and hours of practice, these parents often voice how overwhelming it feels on the day of discharge. *Preemie Care* will be an invaluable resource for families as they navigate that complicated first year."

JEANNE SCOTLAND

RN, MN, neonatal nurse practitioner, Calgary

"A powerful, well-written book with heartfelt stories and excellent data from incredibly educated authors. This is a must-read for any parent or family member dealing with a NICU experience. This book brought tears to our eyes, as nothing is off limits and the content is raw and invaluable."

HEATHER AND JASON MANNA

parents of twenty-nine-week twin boys

"After reading *Preemie Care*, I am more confident. This book has taught me about everything I need to know when my baby comes home and while still in the NICU. One of the most interesting things this book reminded me is to take care of myself, which I had completely forgotten. Being a first-time mom of a twenty-five-weeker, *Preemie Care* was my life saver. One handy source to all my worries as a preemie mom."

DHANVEER KAUR

mother of twenty-five-week son

"This book is an amazing tool for your first year with your preemie. If you can't have Karen or Tammy in your home every week, this is the next best thing."

MICHELLE AND CRAIG HEYNEN

parents of twenty-five-week twin boys

"Leaving the NICU we had no experience with taking care of a baby, much less a preemie. This book wasn't available at that time, but it would have made a huge difference, because it is imbued with the patience and knowledge of its authors and gives so much information about what to expect and what to do in order to take care of your little one."

BIBI

mother of twenty-seven-week daughter

"This book is a must-have for every preemie parent preparing for discharge from the NICU. Too many of us have walked the halls in those final days and hours prior to discharge, wishing we could bring home one of our nurses. This is a great way to do exactly that. Well done!"

DEB DISCENZA

coauthor of *The Preemie Parent's Survival Guide to the NICU* and CEO/publisher of www.preemieworld.com

"This book simplifies the overwhelming and complicated world parents face when they have NICU babies. Using simple language, Karen and Tammy give parents a step-by-step guide from the moment their premature baby is born to the end of the first year at home. It addresses the challenges and also reminds us to celebrate the miracle of life. It's the book every preemie parent has been waiting for."

FABIANA BACCHINI

executive director, Canadian Premature Babies Foundation and author of *From Surviving to Thriving—A Mother's Journey through Infertility, Loss and Miracles*

"As a parent with a baby who's currently in the NICU, this book has given me an inside look into what to expect as we progress through the NICU, as well as the confidence and knowledge to handle any challenges that might arise when I finally get to bring my sweet baby home. An absolute must-read for preemie parenthood!"

SAVANNAH VIKLUND

mother of twenty-six-week son

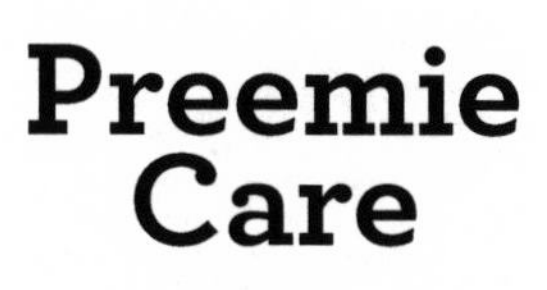
Preemie
Care

Preemie Care

A Guide to Navigating the First Year with Your Premature Baby

Karen Lasby, RN MN CNeoN(C)
and
Tammy Sherrow, RN MN

Foreword by Carole Kenner, PhD RN FAAN FNAP ANEF

Preemie Care

ISBN 978-1-9990443-0-5 (paperback)
ISBN 978-1-9990443-1-2 (ebook)

Produced by Page Two
www.pagetwo.com

Cover design by Teresa Bubela
Interior design by Setareh Ashrafologhalai
Illustrations by Kaylie Sauverwald

The information in this book is not intended as a substitute for the medical care and advice of your baby's health care team. Approaches to preemie health care vary widely across NICUs and countries. Talk to your baby's doctor or pediatrician before changing the plan of care. Information and advice in this book was supported by available evidence at the time of printing. Statements are the opinions of the authors.

www.preemiecare.ca

This book is dedicated to the thousands of preemies and their parents with whom we have walked the preemiehood journey. The capacity, persistence, and love of parents is inspiring.

CONTENTS

FOREWORD

TODAY, SMALLER and sicker babies are surviving and thriving. Yet for families, the homecoming can be as traumatic as the birth of a baby requiring NICU care. For more than thirty years I have been involved in transition from hospital to home research and unfortunately, I hear many of the same parental stories today that I heard when I began this journey. Despite our advances in technology and our follow-up programs, parents still find themselves afloat with many, many questions and fears as they leave the safe NICU environment. Fears about their parenting skills, their ability to recognize if their baby is sick, how to feed their baby, and how to promote positive development are present in the initial months at home and for many families these remain through the baby's first year.

This book, while aimed at parents, will help health professionals understand what it is like to parent a baby in the NICU and then take the baby home. Weathering the storm really does describe the rough entry into and navigation through the NICU. Encouraging parents to care for themselves is something often forgotten in the discharge process. The authors, Karen Lasby and Tammy Sherrow, experts in the neonatal field, really provide parents with information that is essential during that first year. The book follows the journey a parent will take with their baby. Information is offered in chunks with section headings that make finding the content quick and easy. Inclusion of exemplars from parent focus groups makes the content come to life, and feel real to the reader. Parents can relate to these quotations. The final section offering success stories gives parents the encouragement they need to feel they can do this.

Preemie Care fills a gap in neonatal care domestically and globally. Parents cannot provide care to their baby if they are not cared for or feel they can succeed. This book empowers parents and helps the health professional to understand how to ensure that families are part of the care team both inside and outside the NICU. This essential content will support families as they transition from hospital to home and to primary care. The first year is a roller coaster but with *Preemie Care* the ride will be smoother.

CAROLE KENNER
PhD, RN, FAAN, FNAP, ANEF,
president/CEO Council of International
Neonatal Nurses, Inc. (COINN)

INTRODUCTION
An Unexpected Journey

YOUR BABY was born premature. This was an unexpected beginning. You may be feeling confused, overwhelmed, sad, anxious, angry, or guilty. You may be unsure about where you are headed or where you will end up, as though you were "lost at sea." The seas may be rough for both premature babies and parents. Although each family's experience is unique, families face many of the same themes and concerns. Every parent yearns for information, support, guidance, and a competent health care team. Taking home a premature baby can be challenging, frightening, and exhausting. This book serves as a guide for parents to successfully navigate the unknown waters of prematurity during the first year. Although we can't promise turbulence-free waters on your journey, we can assure you that following the advice in this book will help calm those seas.

First, we'd like to congratulate you on the birth of your baby. Welcome to preemiehood! Preterm birth is on the rise in most countries and average nearly one in ten births worldwide. Premature babies are not simply small full-term babies. They need special care to support their growth and development. In the neonatal intensive care unit (NICU) and at home, parents of premature babies often experience challenges. They describe a lack of knowledge and confidence to care for their baby and are unsure about who to turn to for answers.

We wrote this book to provide guidance and support to parents during their journey with their premature baby. Through our experience of caring for more than two thousand premature babies and their families in the NICU and community, we know that so many have been on the same journey that you are on and that they felt relief when they had the support of neonatal nurses along the way. Families we have met over the years have fueled our passion to be highly informed caregivers and teachers. Helping families has been extremely gratifying for us, and many suggested that we write a book so that even more families could access our observations, insight, and expertise.

This book includes information on the NICU experience, preparing for discharge and transitioning home, as well as everyday common issues of prematurity during the first year at home. We offer you many strategies for care so that you and your baby can have the best possible health outcomes.

This book is packed with parent-tested, nurse-designed, and research-informed strategies. We hope you and your baby will benefit from every suggestion. You may wish to read this book from cover to cover. While your baby is in the NICU, we highly recommend that you read the first two chapters, which are designed to help you thrive in the NICU and facilitate your baby's smooth transition home. After you read the first two chapters, you may want to read the chapters in sequence. Or you may want to dip into sections that address your questions, pick and choose, depending on your baby's and family's challenges. The table of contents and index will help you locate the information you're looking for.

Please visit our website, www.preemiecare.ca for additional resources, bonus material, and links to reliable and valuable content. Here we offer educational resources such as newsletters, videos, webinars, and opportunities to connect with us. Follow us on our social media channels: Facebook, Instagram, LinkedIn, and YouTube.

We have been blessed to work with ten families who assisted in the development of this book. Through initial focus groups, these families helped develop the content, and they have provided their powerful, rich stories to make the book come alive. We hope that you can relate to what other parents have gone through and realize that you are not alone in this journey.

♥

Being pregnant was like planning an exciting vacation. We knew our lives would change in November and we wanted to be ready. We picked up pregnancy magazines and started looking into baby furniture and supplies. I watched what I ate and tried to stay active and well rested. Our family and friends were curious about how I was doing and kept asking how far along the pregnancy was. I loved the attention!

And then the unthinkable happened. I started bleeding and was rushed to the hospital. The doctor told me I was already dilated and I would be delivering early. They put me on bed rest and drugs to stop labor. I was also given a drug to speed up my baby's lung development. As I laid there, every twinge and cramp piqued my anxiety. This couldn't be happening to me! I did everything right to have a healthy pregnancy. Why me? Our world was spinning out of control.

One week later we heard that the baby was not doing well and needed to be delivered early. We cried and held one another as I was prepped for surgery. Moments later we caught a glimpse of our baby before they whisked her wet, red, tiny body to the warmer. A team of nurses and doctors swarmed her. In the hours before we were able to see her again, my husband and I were in shock. This all happened so quickly. Our heads were spinning and our hearts pounding. We felt helpless and powerless. Our baby dream had come crashing down.

The NICU sights and sounds were overwhelming. It was hard to concentrate. They used strange abbreviations like RDS, PDA, CPAP, and "A's and B's," and words that made no sense to us, like "saturation," "bradys," and "indrawing." We felt as though we were in a strange land, lost and unsure how to get through this. We saw many other families in the NICU and would lock eyes and nod with compassion. We were all in the same boat.

WEATHERING THE STORM
You and Your Baby in the NICU

GIVING BIRTH is an adventure unlike any other life experience. Most parents anticipate the big event with a mixture of excitement and apprehension. Yet few are truly prepared for any complications that may result in preterm birth or your baby requiring intensive care. When things don't go as planned, you face a more stressful beginning than most parents. Landing in the NICU can be frightening, initially. The unfamiliar sights and sounds can be downright scary. But rest assured that the equipment is there to give your baby the best possible start in life. You will discover a whole new world with its own language and routines.

Not only are you concerned about your baby's health and survival, but you may feel overwhelmed and out of place. In time, you will get to know the people caring for your baby, develop valuable relationships with them, sort out your own role in caring for your baby, and become a part of this new community.

This chapter focuses on this initial experience in the NICU and how you can best care for yourself and your baby during your stay. So often the focus at this point is on the baby and it can be difficult to find your role in the NICU. Many parents say that, months later, once they were home, they realized that their time in the NICU had been traumatic. The research-informed and parent-tested strategies in this chapter will help to ensure that you not only survive but can thrive while in the NICU.

In the blink of an eye, she was outside me. She was supposed to stay for another four months, but there she was. I only saw her for a few seconds. They tell me she is doing well, but I can't see her. I can't touch her. She only weighs a pound. What did I do wrong? Did I cause her early birth? Being in the NICU was the scariest, most terrifying place we had ever been . . . but also the most loving, supportive, amazing place that ever existed.

The NICU journey will affect each family differently. The sudden shock of having a premature baby hits parents in various ways. It is an unexpected beginning. Some parents are in disbelief and have trouble accepting the reality of preterm birth. Some parents react with tears and anxiety. For some parents, the NICU high-tech care reassures them that their baby is getting the best care possible, whereas others are overwhelmed by the equipment and medical language. Some parents draw into themselves, while others reach out for help. All these reactions are normal.

It took me a long time to get comfortable just being in the NICU. The nurse and doctors did their best, but the urgency of that place was extremely overwhelming. Try to remember that the doctors and nurses are there to support you, too. They have seen hundreds of people and reactions in this situation. I found that, once I started to talk about my feelings of insecurity, the nurses were really good at responding in a completely non-judgmental way.

Guilt and feelings of responsibility will cross your mind. You will reflect on your health and pregnancy, searching for answers to a possible cause. Most likely, you will not find anything conclusive. The causes of preterm birth are largely unknown. Nevertheless, it is normal for parents to feel guilty.

Anger may surface. Anger that your birth experience did not go as planned, at your family and friends for not understanding, at your partner for not giving you the support you feel you deserve or even at your baby for coming too soon.

Exhaustion can occur, especially in the early days. Mothers may still be recovering from labor and delivery and now have to cope with the stresses of the NICU. Until you get into a routine life can be a bit chaotic and fatigue can set in.

There will be uncertainty. In the NICU, you may feel like a ship on rocky seas; the journey full of ups and downs. Your days will likely be defined by how well your baby is doing. Most babies have challenging days and those provoke a lot of stress and uncertainty for parents because they worry about the future and potential complications. Some days you will feel comfortable, happy, content. On other days, feelings of sadness, helplessness, and frustration may surface. Positive progress is invigorating and setbacks are hard to take.

♥

My initial experience in the NICU was totally overwhelming; pods of incubators, machines, wires, tubes, beeping, and alarms, people in full scrubs, impossibly tiny babies. I spent hours just sitting beside my son's incubator, staring at him and crying. I experienced a huge mix of intense emotions from love and wonder to fear, sadness, grief, and guilt. As time went by, I got used to the NICU and I began to sort through my feelings. I learned that his time on the NICU would be a roller-coaster experience, and that two steps forward would often be followed by one step back. As difficult as that was, it also taught me to slow down, accept that my son was the boss, and live from moment to moment with him in a mindful way.

Birth of a premature baby raises feelings of loss. You have lost the ideal of the full-term baby and the usual post-birth excitement. You might not receive the traditional post-birth flowers and congratulatory remarks. Instead, you may feel fear, uncertainty, panic, loss of control. You might hold off sending birth announcements. You are not sure if you should share photographs. Family and friends often don't know how to interact with you, for example, should they congratulate you or express sympathy for having a fragile newborn? Often, they do nothing for fear your baby will not survive. The loss of these norms may leave you feeling empty.

Initially, you may be confused about your role in the NICU. Parents often feel separated from their baby and are unsure of how or where they can help. Intimidating equipment such as incubators, monitors, and pumps can erect a physical wall between you and your baby. You may even feel jealous of the way the nurses seem to be able to meet your baby's every need. If your baby is seriously ill, you may worry that your baby could die. This may hold you back from engaging with your baby and complicate feelings of attachment.

Sadness may emerge. The "baby blues" are experienced by approximately 80 percent of mothers within the first few days after birth. Symptoms may include mood swings, crying, worrying, irritability, feelings of helplessness, sadness, anxiety, and difficulty sleeping. In most cases, these symptoms improve or resolve on their own within a week or two and do not require treatment. However, if these symptoms last for more than two weeks or significantly affect your ability to carry out daily activities, you may be experiencing depression. See chapter 7 for more detail about postpartum depression (PPD).

Your baby is in good hands. While this experience can be overwhelming to new parents, try to take comfort in knowing that the majority of babies who require intensive care at birth have excellent outcomes. Rest assured that the team caring for your baby (doctors, nurses, respiratory therapists, dietitians) wants only the best for him or her. They are highly trained and will make use of specialized equipment and technology to ensure the best possible outcome for your baby. Get to know the people caring for your baby. You are a valued member of the team and are so important to your baby's health and future. The learning curve is steep, but you'll get there! Trust the team and lean on them for guidance, information, and support. In a very short time, you will feel more comfortable with this strange and wonderful NICU world.

The NICU is a place that you can't understand until you live it. It can be scary and intimidating, but miracles happen behind those locked doors. The NICU team go to the ends of the earth to protect your vulnerable baby and support your family as much as they can.

This chapter is divided into two sections: Caring for Yourself, and Caring for Your Baby. Together, these will help you navigate the NICU journey.

Caring for Yourself

Many parents feel guilty about taking care of themselves. It is not selfish to pay attention to your needs. You need to take care of yourself so that you have the energy to care for your baby.

> ♥ *Parents in the NICU are often self-critical and take on blame undeservingly. Be mindful of your self-talk and try to be gentle and kind with yourself. Balance out anxiety and negative feelings with a little bit of hope and optimism. If that is too hard some days, remind yourself that you will get through whatever happens.*

Everyone handles the stress of the NICU in their own way. Give yourself time to get used to this new reality. Take life day by day, be kind to yourself, and know this emotional roller coaster is temporary. You will ride through it! Don't blame yourself. You may feel out of control. Accept this for now. As you spend more time in the NICU you will start to feel more confident.

Journal

Consider creating two journals: one to record your baby's journey and one for your private reflections.

Leave your baby's journal at your baby's bedside. Record your visits. Your baby's NICU team can contribute their thoughts and wishes. This will be an amazing keepsake for your baby.

For yourself, buy a nice book to record your thoughts, feelings, worries, joys, and triumphs. This is not your baby's day-by-day journey, but YOUR journey. Start with exploration of your deepest thoughts about the birth and NICU experience. Writing should be free-flow; don't worry about spelling, punctuation, or grammar. This book is for you and is not intended for sharing. Explore why you care about what happened during the day and whether there's an action you need to take. Whenever you experience an emotional event, try to journal about it. The purpose of reflective journaling is to acknowledge the emotional event and recognize the impact on you.

Today was not a good day. She was having a bunch of apneas so they put her back on oxygen. I am so disappointed. I thought we were going home this weekend. What can I do? Nothing. But then I thought I could do something. She loves kangaroo care and her oxygen always goes down. So I held her for an extra-long time and talked to her about hanging in there. I wasn't giving up on her and she shouldn't, either.

Connect with other parents in the NICU

You might not have the energy to start connecting right after your baby is admitted to the NICU. But as soon as you feel comfortable, introduce yourself to other parents to help you gain a sense of community and belonging. Meet up for breaks in the NICU parent room or hospital cafeteria. Go for walks together. Share your contact information.

It was unbelievably helpful to learn that I wasn't the only one having a rough time. Sometimes you just need to talk to another parent who's been there. She reassured me and gave me hope.

Many parents report that these connections were valuable even after their babies were transferred to different hospitals and discharged home.

Try to connect with the other parents. They will understand what you mean when you talk about oxygen saturation or CPAP levels. They may become lifelines for you, even after you go home. We met lifelong friends in the NICU and are grateful that our babies will grow up together.

Ask your baby's nurse about parent support groups or whether the hospital has a one-on-one peer support program. Search for online parent support groups. Some parents find Facebook groups for preemie parents to be helpful, whereas others find these resources overwhelming. If you are interested in connecting with other parents on Facebook, see our website at www.preemiecare.ca. Assistance from previous NICU parents is effective in helping new parents feel "normal" and in navigating the NICU experience.

Take care of yourself physically

To maintain your energy and health, you need adequate sleep, hydration, and nutrition. Often parents neglect their health as they focus on the baby. But this is not sustainable in the long term.

♥ *I created basic routines in my day by keeping regular mealtimes. I packed lunch and snacks every morning before heading to the NICU and used those meals as breaks to relax, get perspective, and recharge. This basic structure in my day was easy to maintain and helped me to feel more in control. I also needed to eat very regularly because pumping took a lot out of me. If I did not eat, I could not produce as much milk and I felt faint, which in turn made it more difficult for me to handle the stress of everything.*

ACTION PLAN: Healthy Eating

Try these strategies for healthy eating:

- Eat regular meals. Plan your meals a day or two in advance so that you don't miss meals or eat less optimal choices (such as junk food).
- Eat nutrient-dense foods. Get protein at each meal, healthy carbohydrates (vegetables, fruit) and healthy fats (avocados, nuts, fatty fish, olive oil).
- Make extra when you prepare a meal so that you have leftovers.
- Use your support network to provide meals that you can store in your freezer. Ask if your NICU has any meals or snacks for parents.
- Minimize your fast-food intake. Although these meals are convenient, they do not provide optimal nutrition.

- If you can afford it, purchase healthy prepared meals.
- If pumping or breastfeeding, ensure you eat enough and drink sufficient water.
- You do not need to avoid any foods if you are making breast milk. Many medicines taken by mothers are safe for breastfeeding, but check with your nurse or doctor about the medications you are taking, including over-the-counter medications. Avoid illicit drugs, cannabis, and alcohol.

♥ *It may feel overwhelming to try to do everything people suggest for self-care. You need a healthy body to remain present for your baby and family. Each day, plan to do one or two simple things that you can achieve easily. Prioritize what is important to you, for example, showering, walking the dog, packing lunch and snacks for the NICU. Each night, reflect on what worked and what didn't. Don't beat yourself up if you didn't meet your goals. Tomorrow is another day.*

Provide breast milk

Research has shown that survival and overall health for premature or sick newborns are improved if babies are given breast milk early and exclusively. Premature babies are less likely to develop infections, chronic lung disease, or necrotizing enterocolitis (NEC), and have better vision and brain development outcomes. Breast milk enhances feed tolerance through its enzymes and growth factors so babies who receive breast milk have fewer feeding interruptions and can advance to full feeds earlier. Not to mention the cost savings to you, as formula is expensive!

Even if you were not originally planning to breastfeed, you might choose to provide breast milk while your baby is small and fragile. That would be an amazing gift to your baby. Women who deliver prematurely make breast milk that is higher in anti-inflammatory and nutritional value. If you are not able to provide breast milk, there may be donor human milk available. Even a short course of breast milk can have a positive impact on your baby's health and development.

I overheard a conversation with a health care provider and a mom about how to balance life while pumping for her baby in the NICU, with a young child at home, and post C-section. In that moment, I realized that what's asked of new NICU moms is nearly impossible. Do your best to be kind to yourself. Your baby needs a functioning, healthy mother to advocate for them, too. It helped me to commit to pumping one day at a time so that I didn't get overwhelmed by the idea of pumping for months. I'm now at almost sixteen months and going strong.

The decision to continue pumping or breastfeeding after the NICU is totally yours. You will find more information about breastfeeding in chapter 4.

ACTION PLAN: Breast Milk Pumping

Try these strategies for early breast milk pumping:

- Remove milk regularly to give your breast a clear message to produce more. The expressed volume will be very low at first but will build. Every drop counts!
- Ask a NICU nurse or lactation consultant about how often and how to massage and hand-express milk from your breasts.
- Ask for a syringe or small cup to capture your first drops of milk. These precious drops of colostrum are very important for your baby's immunity.
- While in the hospital, learn to use the electric pumps. Ask for advice about the correct size flange. You don't want it to rub and irritate your nipple or to be so loose that the pump doesn't create enough suction. Learn how to adjust the suction pressure. The suction should not be painful.
- Rent a commercial breast pump for at home. A "hospital grade" breast pump most effectively supports breast milk production. Good pumps can be costly, so check with your health insurance plan and research the best rates. You may want to compare rental costs against the cost to purchase. If you buy secondhand, purchase new tubing.
- Save time by pumping both breasts at the same time ("double pumping").

- Massage your breasts with your hands while you pump. A warm cloth may soften the ducts before pumping.
- Every time you pump, sit back, relax, and drink a glass of water.
- Bring a picture of your baby or an item of baby clothing to help you visualize and relax.
- Pump at least seven to eight times a day. Set your clock at night for at least one pump between 1 a.m. and 6 a.m. During this time period, you produce the most prolactin, which promotes breast milk production.
- Keep a package of labels and a pen handy so you can label your milk with the date.
- After pumping, cover your pumped milk and place it in the fridge. You can combine chilled milk and freeze it in larger bottles.
- If you are freezing milk in plastic bags, place the bags in a box so that the bags are not accidentally punctured in your freezer.
- Use a deep freezer for long-term storage of breast milk, if possible. Fridge freezers have limited storage time because they are opened more frequently.
- Use the oldest breast milk first.
- Carefully follow the instructions for cleaning the parts of the pump and bottles.
- Monitor your production. Your milk supply will progress from a few drops to larger quantities over time. Within a couple of weeks, you will produce over 500 ml (17 oz.). If you do not yield 500 ml/day, contact your baby's nurse and a lactation consultant. There are natural and medicinal products that may help with lactation.
- Consult your baby's nurse or the NICU lactation consultant for further guidance.

Ride the emotional roller coaster

Many people experience emotional ups and downs and it is okay to not feel like yourself in the NICU. The waves of uncertainty are a big part of the NICU journey. Uncertainty will spike when your baby has setbacks and will settle with improvements. Mothers and fathers report feeling stress during the NICU stay. It is okay to cry, express frustration, or feel angry. If your emotions boil over, step away from the situation, take a break, and reach out for support.

> ♥ *I became so protective over my son's progress that any little perceived setback was devastating. I worried that there was something the doctors weren't telling me (which I logically knew was not true) or that there was some major health concern being missed. I must have been told about two hundred times, "We will just keep an eye on it." That was frustrating because I felt I couldn't handle another ounce of uncertainty. Waiting for answers and outcomes and living with uncertainty was the hardest part, by far, for me.*

Worrying about the present and future is normal. Consider that no parent really knows what the future will hold for their child. However, stress and worry should not overwhelm you. Try to accept the uncertainty and "roll with it." You can't undo the uncertainty by worrying about it. You'll just exhaust yourself. You will learn from experience that you can manage the uncertainty and it will in turn become less stressful.

> ♥ *It was extremely overwhelming to think that we might need to spend four months in the NICU. That is what can happen when your baby is born at twenty-four weeks. We had to look at the small picture, prioritize what was really important, and live one day at a time. That allowed us to be more present, not only for our daughter but also for ourselves. We started to deal with our baby's health issues in a more positive way. Our mantra was, "Every day, great victories." If she lived for another day, despite all complications, it was a really good day!*

ACTION PLAN: Easing Stress

Try these strategies to ease the stress of uncertainty:

- Take it one day at a time.
- Identify one strength of your baby every day.
- Journal about the highs and lows.
- Reflect on the positive progress to date.
- Keep the possibilities in the foreground and the problems in the background.
- Practice patience.
- Distract yourself.
- Seek information and advice.
- Surround yourself with helpful supports.

Clarify health coverage

Investigate how and when to add your baby(s) to your health benefit plan. The earlier you do this, the better. In some areas, the addition of your baby(s) to your health benefit plan should occur within thirty days of birth to avoid a financial cost. Contact your health benefit provider and request information in writing. Be sure to write down notes about these conversations (with date, name of person you spoke to, and outcome of conversation). If you don't have health insurance, contact the hospital social worker as soon as possible.

Do you have options for maternity and/or critical illness benefits? How can you best use your maternity benefits, paternity benefits, and/or unemployment benefits? Find out the eligibility for critical illness benefits for families. Ask your health care insurance company about whether they cover specialty medications, formula, or breast pumps. Again, write notes about these conversations. The social worker in the NICU may guide you to where to get more information.

Connect with family, friends, and coworkers

Your support people will want to know what's happening. And you will want to share your happy and sad feelings with them. You will want to celebrate when your baby comes off the ventilator or when you hold your baby for the first time or when your baby no longer needs oxygen. But phone and email communications take a lot of time and energy.

♥ *We come from big families and have lots of relatives in other countries. Everyone kept asking, When are we getting a picture of him? What's happening now? How big is he? I barely had enough time to shower and eat. How could I possibly answer all their messages? I knew they cared, but I was in survival mode.*

♥ *Think about who you need most right now. This is the person or people to stay in contact with. I picked one friend and one family member as my "go-to" people. I knew my mom would share with the rest of the family. And my girlfriend was someone I could confide in. When I took time to talk, text, or email these two people, I knew it was for me as much as it was for them.*

To save time, communicate with family and friends through an online shareable platform, such as a Google document, personal blog, closed Facebook group, or group distribution list for email or texting. Or use a phone app such as WhatsApp.

♥ *At first it was hard to share pictures, videos, and the details surrounding our son's early arrival. However, once we took the leap of faith and shared his journey, it was extremely reassuring to know how many people we had cheering us on.*

Connect with professional supports

Ask your baby's nurse about available supports, such as social workers, psychologists, physicians, and parent support programs. If you are from out of town, ask about nearby accommodations and resources.

♥

Many times, we were caught in critical situations that required a lot of us, but we were too fragile to think straight. Making decisions on behalf of someone who cannot speak up for herself can be extremely painful and scary. When we did not know what to do, we talked to a psychologist and found a couple of people on the team with whom we could speak more freely. That is how we got a better picture of the real situation and made the best choices for our baby.

Talk to someone if you are struggling in any way. It is normal to be anxious, overwhelmed, or sad when your baby is not doing well. Be concerned about your mental health if your baby is doing better and your mood does not change to reflect that. Please take care of yourself. Asking for help is not a sign of weakness. In fact, it shows great personal strength and courage.

♥

I thought my anxiety was normal and that it would go away with time. But it wasn't until months after the NICU and life was settling that I could turn the mirror on myself and see that I was not okay. I needed help. My doctor connected me right away. I wish I had done this when my baby was in the NICU.

If you do not get help with prolonged symptoms, your mental health and happiness are at risk, not to mention the negative impact on parent-baby attachment and your baby's development. These may be common after a traumatic birth or NICU experience, but should not be ignored. Please refer to chapter 7 for more information on postpartum depression (PPD) and post-traumatic stress disorder (PTSD).

Seek helping hands

Parents report exhaustion when trying to balance NICU and home responsibilities. Seek and accept help offered from family, friends, and community members. It can be hard to ask for help or explain what you need. When people ask what they can do for you while your baby is in the NICU, instead of saying "nothing," gratefully accept their offer and suggest frozen or takeout meals, errands, rides to and from the hospital to avoid parking fees, care for older children, yard care, and so on. Explain what you need. Rely on support people who actually *help* and do not add to your burden. It is best not to have people visit at this time unless they are helpful.

♥ *I thought I could do it by myself. After all, it was only one baby. But I was losing it. The travel was killing me. I was trying to pump regularly and take milk to the hospital and keep up with meals and laundry and all that home stuff. Where could I fit in sleeping or eating? It was tough for us to ask for and accept help. My husband and I are immigrants and we have always taken care of our lives without asking for anyone's help. However, we learned to lean on our closest family and friends and we asked the social worker for help. Ask for help, accept it, and do not feel bad about it.*

Go to www.preemiecare.ca to download a letter that you can edit and share with your family and friends:

Dear loved one,

I am going through a challenging and scary time. Spending time in the hospital is isolating and exhausting. Here are some ways that you could help:

- Visit me at the hospital because it is difficult for me to leave my baby for long. I might not have the energy or time to have company at home.
- Do not visit me if you have any symptoms of illness or if you have been looking after anyone who is ill. I cannot get sick. Babies in the NICU are very fragile and cannot be exposed to germs.
- Be flexible and understanding. Things can change quickly in the NICU and I may suddenly be unavailable because my baby is having a bad day or I'm having a hard time coping.
- Understand that likely you are not going to see the baby; most NICUs have strict policies about who can visit.
- Make food for me that can be frozen and eaten later. If I'm not home, you could give it to another close friend or family member who can get it to me.

- Treat me to a coffee or a meal, even better if it is homemade or bought outside the hospital.
- Buy me a gift card for restaurants in or close to the hospital.
- Take care of some of the everyday things in my life that I may not have time for right now, such as housecleaning, laundry, feeding or walking the dog, looking after or entertaining my other children.
- Ask how my baby is doing that particular day. Things can change moment to moment and certainly day to day for babies in the NICU, so asking how my baby is doing in general is too big a question for me to answer.
- Ask to see pictures of my baby and show an interest in my baby beyond his/her medical condition. Having a baby is exciting and parents in the NICU have little opportunity to show off their new bundle.
- Look up some images of NICU babies online before you visit so you know what to expect.
- Don't take it personally if I don't want or have time to talk. I appreciate that you care.
- Most importantly, BE THERE for ME. Offer me a listening ear or shoulder to cry on. You don't have to have the perfect thing to say, just be there for me. You don't have to do anything necessarily, just show me you care.
- I apologize if I forget to thank you or respond to you.
- Understand that I may not be able to be there for you while my baby is in the NICU. Once things settle down, I want to hear more about your life and be there to support you again.

Thank you from the bottom of my heart. You are my life preserver.

Establish a workable routine

Strike a balance between NICU time and home time. Don't try to be a "super parent" by taking on everything. Some parents have older children at home who need their parents, too! Separation can be hard for young children and may result in separation anxiety and developmental regressions, for example, needing to use diapers again, not staying in bed, wanting a bottle.

♥ *I felt guilty no matter where I was. When I was in the NICU with my twins, I felt guilty about leaving my other daughter and not taking care of my home. When I was at home, I felt guilty about not being with my twins. I couldn't win. I felt torn in all directions. And there is only one of me.*

Communicate with the NICU staff about the needs of your other children. If your toddler is home sick, you should discuss whether to stay home until the toddler is well and you are free from illness, too. Share what is going on in your busy household so the NICU staff understand why your time is limited. Discuss options for childcare with your family and friends to reduce the pressure on you. Can a support person drive your other children to school this month or help with childcare? Are there affordable options in your community, such as half-day daycare? If you do not have any support people, ask to speak to the NICU social worker to discuss options.

Be realistic about what to expect of yourself. Being organized will help you manage your schedule. Try packing a lunch for the NICU and figuring out the best times to be with your baby and when you need to be home. But be flexible enough that you can modify the routine if needed.

Take time away from the NICU

Take time away from the NICU. Parents feel torn between time in the NICU and time away. Permit yourself small breaks, walks, or enjoyable activities to rejuvenate yourself. Ask if your NICU has a parent lounge. Everyone needs an occasional break to keep a positive state of mind.

♥ *If your NICU stay is a longer one, take shifts with family members so that you have a break. Go home to sleep at night, and know that your baby's nurse is a phone call away. As hard as it is, you need to take care of yourself, too.*

Some NICUs may have a place for parents to sleep, either short-term or long-term, near their baby. Staying with your baby in the NICU has been shown to have great advantages, such as reduced infections, shorter time to full feeds, shorter time in hospital, and greater parent confidence. If your baby stays in the NICU for a week or two, staying over might be very manageable. But you will need to go home periodically to take care of laundry, groceries, and your home. Longer NICU stays are hard on parents. Juggling between NICU and home becomes challenging. As much as you'd like to stay in the NICU until your baby comes home, regular life needs your attention, too.

♥ *It took a while to say to myself, It's okay to go home! You have to have faith in the nurses, doctors, and RTS. It is so important to get rest and sleep. It doesn't work without Mom and Dad being healthy and mentally able to cope with whatever comes their way.*

Celebrate milestones

Take regular photographs of your baby and your family. You could try using a consistent item to gauge your baby's growth, such as a teddy bear, your wedding ring, or your phone. Save mementos such as a lock of hair or hospital identification band. Consider hand and footprints. Premature babies have unique milestones to celebrate, such as the first kangaroo care (skin-to-skin) cuddle, 1,000-gram weight achievement, first day off oxygen, first day wearing a sleeper, and first breastfeed. Since you missed out on the tradition of sending out birth announcements, you could choose one of these special moments to share your pride and joy. Design your own milestone certificate using the template you can download from our website at www.preemiecare.ca.

♥ *Celebrate the little successes. Every hour, every day, your baby is one step closer to going home. Stand back and see how incredibly strong your tiny human is. In my eyes, my daughter is the strongest person I have ever met. She is my biggest hero. And she is only thirteen months old. Not many people can say that. NICU babies are a special kind of miracle.*

Help your partner

The NICU is hard on relationships. Couples struggle to keep communication lines open and support one another. Your time is limited. Responsibilities and stress are high. Often one parent must return to work.

Interactions between couples may be affected when they have different styles of coping and communicating. One partner might assume the strong supportive role. One partner may be quieter or not able to verbalize their true feelings as easily as the other partner. Some partners use emotional or communicative ways to cope with their stress. Some are quick to respond to situations and others need time to reflect on information before making decisions. Couples need to appreciate the strengths of their partner.

Try to incorporate both parents in the journey. So often support is available for mothers, but fathers are often on the sidelines. Dads feel the emotional instability as much as moms, so make sure you are both getting the support you need.

> ♥ *My partner was a talker and crier. And I needed to be the rock. I asked the questions so we knew what was happening. I couldn't lose it. At least not in front of anyone.*

Make time as a couple to check in with one another using the "partner conversation starters" below. Take time to truly listen. Acknowledge one another's feelings.

Partner conversation starters:

"Are you doing okay?"

"What do you think about our baby's setback today?"

"I'm feeling really stressed about our baby. I need ideas. How do you handle your stress?"

"You've been really quiet today. What's on your mind?"

"We could really use a break from all this stress we are under. Do you have any ideas?"

"I'm feeling exhausted today. Can you help me with dinner so we can both go to the NICU tonight?"

Couples also find that their time is fully booked between NICU trips, work, and home responsibilities. Plan together to carve out some time for one another. Expect that sexual relations will be temporarily dampened by the stress. In the meantime, spend quality time together to maintain your cohesive unit.

> *I very much looked forward to the evenings and weekends in the NICU because I could be there with my partner. We used the time to catch up and connect. It really helped with my stress levels and solidified our relationship. We also started pizza Fridays, the one evening we would eat at the hospital cafeteria together; it kicked off the weekend on a more relaxed note.*

For some couples, enduring a hardship makes the relationship stronger. Couples that pull together as a unit are more resilient to life stressors.

Explore your spirituality

Cultural, spiritual, and religious beliefs may bring you comfort and help you to feel less stressed during your NICU stay. Having a belief in something bigger than your immediate experience can be a powerful stress buffer. When you feel part of a greater whole, you may realize that you are not responsible for everything that happens in life.

At the same time, it's normal for this experience to challenge your religious and spiritual beliefs. You might feel angry that this happened to you and question your faith. Talk to your religious leaders about your turmoil and how your faith can help you during your time of need.

Meditation, quiet reflection, and prayer can be relaxing and calming, and ultimately re-energizing.

> *I found a beautiful little non-denominational chapel in the hospital where I could be alone with my thoughts. I could pray. I could gather myself. Sometimes I just needed some quiet time away from the busy NICU.*

Seek support from your religious or spiritual community and cultural groups. You may find comfort speaking with a pastor, priest, rabbi, minister, elder, or imam. The hospital pastoral service may be helpful for families who are away from home or spending a lot of time in the hospital. Many hospitals also have a multicultural department to help families include their cultural customs, rituals, or ceremonies for peace, comfort, and strength with having a fragile baby in hospital.

♥ *It does not matter what your beliefs are, or if you do not believe in anything at all. NICU will show that science can only go so far, and that some babies do not follow what is written in the books and have very different outcomes, despite the same protocol and treatment. After everything our baby went through, she was supposed to have many problems and she was not even supposed to be alive. But she was. Love and faith can do great things along with science. You do not have to choose one or the other; let them hold hands, pray or hope for the best, and you will see that unexplainable things happen.*

Leaning on your cultural, spiritual, or religious support system can lend emotional strength and hope, and can guide you through this challenging time. Taking care of yourself is not selfish. In order to weather the NICU storm and to be there for your baby, you need to be strong, both physically and emotionally.

♥ *Some days you will feel strong, optimistic... other days you will be in pieces, unsure of how you will ever make it through. Be kind to yourself. It is okay to feel this way. You WILL make it through. The experience will change you, but you will likely find yourself feeling grateful for the experience and new perspectives.*

Caring for Baby

Parents often feel helpless when their baby is in NICU. Getting informed and involved will foster your confidence and competence in caring for your baby. The sooner you become comfortable, the sooner you will feel powerful as a parent.

Get to know the NICU

The NICU environment is scary for most families and the sights and sounds can be overwhelming. Find out the location of the parent rooms, bathrooms, breast pumps, water fountains. Learn about the routines such as when rounds and shift change occur. Focus on your baby's bedside and the equipment that supports your baby.

> ♥ *Learn what the monitors mean, but, in the back of your mind, remember that soon there will be no monitors and you will have to rely on your strong Mommy or Daddy skills to read your baby.*

Get to know the NICU team. There are a lot of nurses, doctors, respiratory therapists, and dietitians looking after your baby. You won't be able to remember all their names! But you will become familiar with their roles in the care of your baby. Ask if your NICU can arrange for consistency in nursing caregivers. Care consistency will help your baby's progress.

> ♥ *I loved having a team of primary nurses so that I always knew who was looking after my baby, and I could trust that they knew her.*

Get to know the language of the NICU. The staff often use abbreviations for medical issues and treatments, which can seem confusing at first. Some NICUs may have a handout to explain these terms.

Seek information

Knowledge is power and information can help to reduce stress. Be cautious when searching the internet! You will discover both accurate and misleading information. The most reliable websites would be associated with hospitals, universities, or health care professionals. These sites may give you a good overview of health issues related to prematurity. However, this information needs to be verified by your baby's health care team. Parent blogs may contain advice that is not founded in research or may be unsafe.

Write your questions down. Ask "why?" Direct the majority of your questions to the health care team or use the resource library in your NICU or in your hospital, if there is one. Expect to receive conflicting advice from time to time. Seek clarification. Ask as many questions as you need to, as it can be a steep learning curve in the beginning. No question is silly—ask anything. It is better to have a concrete answer from professionals than to guess and end up guessing wrong. Request information in writing so that you can refer to it later. Bring a notebook with you to the NICU to jot down things your nurses and doctors say, and to record questions you have for them.

Request meetings with your partner and your neonatologist or nurse practitioner so that you both hear the update. It can be hard for one parent to accurately share information with another. Sometimes details get missed or misconstrued.

♥ *Get involved during rounds. Ask questions, pose your ideas. The doctors are the experts, but you are your baby's strongest advocate.*

Understand your baby's age

"Chronologic age" is your baby's age as determined by the actual birth date. We celebrate birthdays by using the chronologic age. We use chronologic age to know when to vaccinate babies.

"Corrected age" is your baby's age based on your baby's due date. If your baby is quite premature, health care professionals will use your baby's corrected age (sometimes called adjusted age) when evaluating the baby's growth and development. So if a baby is six months old, but was born two months early, the corrected age is four months.

When your twenty-four-week preterm baby is four months old, they have finally reached their "due date" and we can expect that this baby will act like a term baby, even though, chronologically, they are four months old.

The age of babies born less than thirty-five weeks' gestation should be adjusted for their prematurity. By using your baby's "true" or corrected age, you are essentially giving your baby credit for their degree of prematurity. Corrected age is more important when monitoring the development of babies born more than one month early. If your premature baby was born less than one month early, developmental progress will likely not be greatly impacted by the prematurity.

To calculate your baby's corrected age prior to your due date, add your baby's birth gestational age (actual age out of forty weeks) to the number of weeks since your baby was born. For example, if your baby was born at twenty-four weeks' gestation and is now six weeks old, your baby is thirty weeks corrected age. Your baby is still ten weeks premature.

To calculate corrected age prior to your due date, apply the formula:

birth gestational age + weeks of age = corrected age

therefore

24 weeks' gestation + 2 weeks old = 26 weeks corrected age
33 weeks' gestation + 4 weeks old = 37 weeks

Once your baby has surpassed your due date, calculate your baby's corrected age by subtracting the number of months of prematurity from your baby's age. For example, if your baby's chronologic age is eight months, and your baby was born two months premature, you would subtract the number of months of prematurity from the chronologic age—eight months minus two months is six months corrected age.

8 months since birth date (chronologic age)
– 2 months born early

6 months corrected age

Another strategy is to calculate your baby's corrected age by using your due date. For example, if your due date was January 1 and it is now April 15, your baby's corrected age is two and a half months (fourteen weeks).

Use the following table to calculate your baby's corrected age.

Corrected age calculator

	Example	Your baby
Due date	January 1	
Today's date	April 15	
Difference between these dates	3.5 months (14 weeks)	

Knowing your baby's corrected age will help you understand the language used in the NICU and appreciate your baby's "true" age.

Participate in care

Participating in care gives you opportunities to bond with your baby and get to know your baby's personality, likes and dislikes, and individual cues. Is he active today? Does she have nice big eyes? Does he respond well to your touch? Is she feisty?

Outcomes are best for babies when their parents are able to be active members of the care team.

♥ *Always be hands on with your baby's care, such as diaper change, bath time, temperature check, mouth care, and when appropriate feeding your baby.*

Design special care activities that just you do, such as singing, talking, reading to your baby, "kangaroo care" (also called skin-to-skin care, shown below), breastfeeding, and tender loving touch. In particular, skin-to-skin contact can calm your baby and help with temperature, growth, oxygenation, and sleep. Skin-to-skin care is also beneficial for parents, as it increases breast milk supply, lowers stress, boosts parent confidence, and promotes parent-baby attachment.

♥ *The first time I held my baby girl, I was so scared but bursting with happiness. Happy tears ran down my cheeks and dropped on her. It was the first time I truly felt like a mother.*

Try to do as much skin-to-skin as possible while you are with your baby. It is so good for both of you.

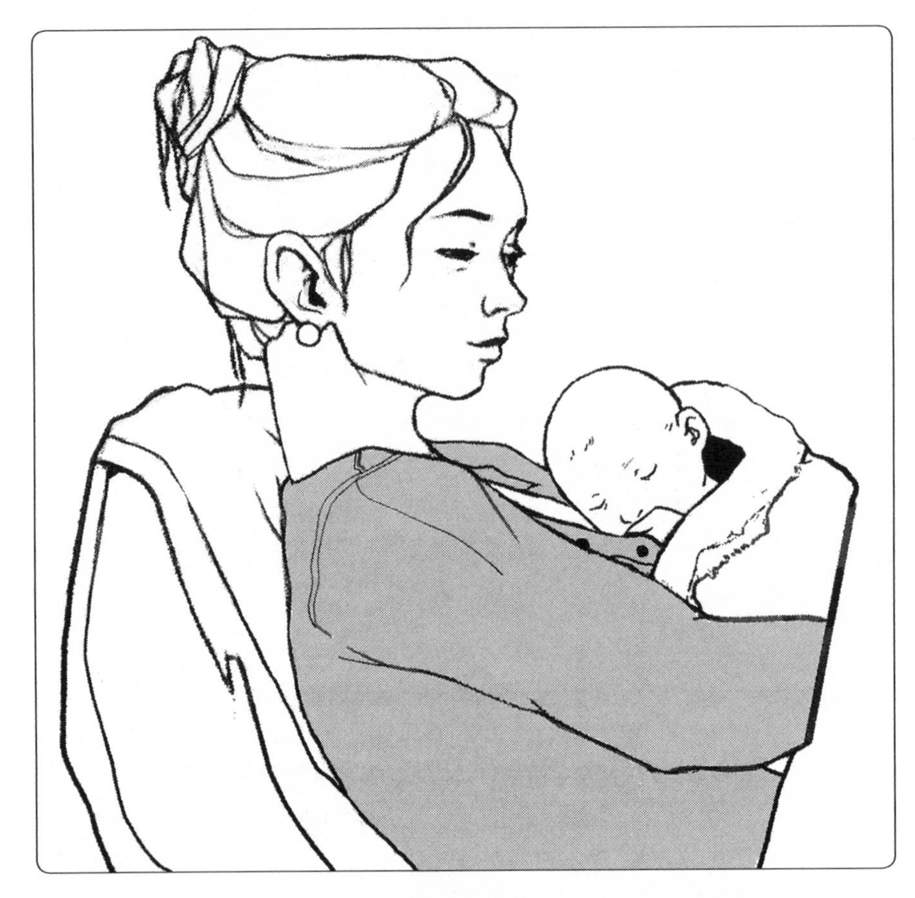

Kangaroo care is skin-to-skin contact with your baby.

♥ *I didn't know dads could do kangaroo care, too. I came in one morning because my wife had the sniffles. I was worried my chest hair would bother my boy, but he just nestled right in and his need for oxygen went way down.*

♥ *We all experience fear differently in the NICU. My husband took a little more time to get involved because he was scared to hurt her, to bond with someone who was not going to stay, or to lose her because of something he had done. He touched one of her feet after almost a month a half, and only held her when she was 1.5 kg (3.3 lbs.). The healthier she got, the braver he became. And look at them now: they are best buddies, reading books together and playing on the floor.*

There may be days when your baby is not stable enough for skin-to-skin care. Talk to your baby's nurse about alternative ways to touch your baby, such as using your hands to surround your baby's body. Your hands will be comforting and containing, like a "bed hug." Your baby will learn the difference between your gentle touch and voice and the therapeutic touch of the staff.

Try to personalize your baby's space. Ask your baby's nurse about bringing items such as pictures, clothing, and cultural or spiritual objects from home. If you do, label them. Don't bring your most cherished items as loss is possible.

Get involved in the feeding process from the beginning, whether that includes giving your baby a soother, helping with tube feedings, offering drops of milk on the lips, working on breast milk supply with regular pumping or bottle feeding. Ask for help from your baby's nurse and lactation consultant. Ask your baby's nurse about feeding routines and strategies. Learn how to read your baby's cues for when to start, stop, or continue feeding.

Be your baby's advocate

As you get to know your baby, you will become your baby's best advocate. You will be able to be their voice to convey what is best for them.

♥ *My baby hated heel pokes. He cried and turned purple. But he was more relaxed if he got heel pokes while we were doing kangaroo care. So I told the nurse to wait till I could get there to hold him.*

You are becoming an expert on your baby. Parents spend more time with their baby than any other member of the health care team and know their baby best. Your input and observations are extremely valuable. Share your knowledge with the NICU staff. Always make your wishes known and trust your instincts. Ask your nurse for a whiteboard or if you can bring in a small one, and write down things you know about your baby that would be helpful for staff to be aware of, so they can be informed even when you are not there.

Enjoy the little moments . . . literally

You are on a completely unique, incredible journey of parenthood, one that will be over before you know it. Take time to appreciate the surprising characteristics of your baby, the amazing achievements of your family, and the special moments to cherish.

♥ *Take the positives or uniqueness and indulge. For example, most parents don't get to see their baby's hair, nails, eyelashes, even nipples grow! Most parents don't know the amazing feeling to see their baby in a onesie for the first time. Most parents don't get to fall completely in love as soon as we did. Sure, we wish it had been different, but it was still good and beautiful.*

Final Thoughts

Although you are going through a lot, know that you can do this, just as countless other parents have. You can adjust to your journey and see the beauty of your new life.

♥ *Our NICU experience started very stressfully, as I went into spontaneous labor when our little bug was only twenty-three weeks and one day. I arrived at the hospital fully dilated and the doctors said that not much could be done other than an emergency C-section. My blood pressure was low and baby was not only breech, but also showing a progressively dropping heart rate. No time for steroid shots, magnesium, or antibiotics; they took me straight to the OR. Our baby came into this world measuring thirty centimeters long and weighing five hundred grams (including plastic wrap, tube, and toque). We were very scared as they took our girl out and we did not hear her crying and were not able to see her right away. After the surgery, we were just grateful that our baby was alive. The doctors had a very serious conversation, first with my husband and then with both of us, about what to expect from a baby born so prematurely. Developmental delays, physical impairments, and a whole life of disabilities, if she managed to stay alive, of course. Giving up on her was not even a possibility, so we agreed that as long as our girl kept fighting, no matter what, we would be at her side, loving her with all our hearts, every day even more. That began our NICU "roller-coaster" ride.*

Our baby made it through the critical window (the first three days) in what they called the "honeymoon phase." Everything was going along wonderfully, but then we started to fall . . . fall very deeply. We cried. A bunch. Every single day. But at the same time, we realized that we had to be strong for her. Our bug faced every problem of prematurity, such as chronic lung disease, feeding intolerance, and retinopathy of prematurity, and a long list of medical complications, including intestine perforation, massive pulmonary hemorrhage, and kidney failure. She faced uncountable pokes and tests and spent time in three NICUs.

We almost lost hope, many times. I still remember the day I arrived home and asked God why He allowed us to put up a nursery if our baby was not coming home. My husband held me and we cried for a long time. After that, we started to do something different. We stopped asking her to stay no matter what. We started telling her that if it was too much suffering, we would be okay if she decided to leave. However, we would love for her to stay, and if she decided to, we would not let her be alone; we would be at her side, always.

She decided to stay. She fought like we've never seen anyone do before. After 155 days in the NICU, we went home. No oxygen, no lines, no feeding tube. Just a tiny baby full of faith and courage, trying to write her own story and experience life with all its beauty. We are witnessing this miracle grow and beat all odds. So far, six months later, she does not show any signs of complications and her growth is progressing very well. And even if there comes a time to deal with a problem, we will do it together, as we did before. She gave us the blessing to be her parents, and that is huge. Since the beginning, it was never about us. It was always about her.

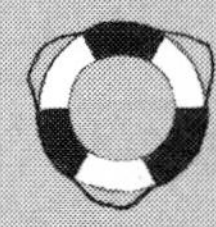

EXPERT TIPS

Here are the key strategies to navigate the journey

- Care for yourself.
- Seek information about your baby.
- Participate in care.
- Get to know your baby.
- Advocate for your baby.
- Use your life preservers (your support network: family, friends, health care professionals).

2

HOMEWARD BOUND
From the NICU to Home

As your baby grows and has fewer medical issues, the time comes to think about going home. The length of your NICU stay can influence your feelings about discharge. A long stay might mean you feel reluctant to let go of your relationship with the staff—or might mean that you are more than ready to go home! The thought of finally bringing baby home fills parents with a mixture of emotions. On the one hand, they are ecstatic to leave the NICU behind. On the other hand, parents are fearful of their ability to assume total care of their baby. All parents of hospitalized newborns will feel some apprehension as discharge nears.

Being prepared will make a big difference to your transition home. The first part of this chapter provides key markers that signal your baby is getting close to discharge and strategies to prepare yourself, your home, your family, and your baby for the big day. This information will help you avoid being caught off guard when the discharge process steps up. The second part of this chapter offers advice for the first few weeks at home. These can be stressful, but our recommendations will help you manage.

♥ *Going home. I'll never forget it. It was the happiest but scariest day. It all started when we spent a night in the care-by-parent room near the NICU. We didn't get much sleep. He wasn't used to the quiet and dark. And we weren't used to anything. We fumbled our way through the night. We were given our walking papers during morning rounds. We were so happy, but so tired. We packed up in record time. The nurses and doctors met us at the reception desk and were so happy for us. Everyone was all smiles.*

And then the moment came when we had to say goodbye. My partner left to warm up the car and park in front of the hospital. So it was up to me to say the final goodbye. How do you say goodbye to your lifeline?

As I turned to walk away, my footsteps felt heavy. It felt as though tethers of support were being torn from my body. My heart was racing and I felt the enormous weight of responsibility for my little baby in the carrier on my arm. Could we do this all by ourselves? Were we ready? So many questions flooded our minds. As I walked toward the car with baby in tow, I promised my son that I would do the best I could.

Pre-Departure

As they say in the NICU, discharge really begins the minute your baby is admitted. In other words, all the care of your baby since birth has been in preparation for discharge. And ever since NICU admission, your baby has been working toward stabilization and the ultimate goal of going home. As we advised in chapter 1, you have been participating in your baby's care. You have been learning about your baby's needs, how your baby communicates, and how to care for your baby. You are getting ready.

Transferring units

When babies mature and grow in the NICU, they will sometimes be transferred to another unit within the same hospital or to a different hospital closer to home. The unit may be called intermediate care, NICU step-down, special care, growing preemie unit, Level II unit, or something else. Whatever it's called, your baby's transfer signals that they have matured beyond the need for intensive life support.

Babies may be transferred to other hospitals for several reasons:

- They are stable, more mature, and no longer require the intensive level of care of the NICU.
- They are no longer on a ventilator but may still need intravenous fluids, oxygen, tube feeds, and medications.
- They do not require specialty care at the current NICU.
- A bed is available at a receiving hospital.
- A bed is available at a hospital closer to home.

Many parents are anxious about transfers and worry that their baby is not ready, may not tolerate the travel, or may not be as well cared for in the new unit/hospital. Even when you know a transfer means your baby is doing better, the transition can be stressful. You are leaving the unit and staff that you have come to know and trust. Additionally, sometimes the decision to transfer is made quickly and without much notice.

Rest assured that the health care team will make the best decisions for your baby. They will transfer your baby to a unit that is equipped to care for their specific needs. Your baby's current health care team will discuss their condition with the future team and share all the important information.

You may feel a little out of sorts when you get to the new unit, which will have different routines and staff. Once you become familiar with the unit, you will settle in again. When you move closer to home or to a unit that is less intense or hectic, it is often possible to relax more and really get to know your baby. Both you and your baby will find it calmer in a unit with less hustle and bustle. Here you will become more directly involved in your baby's care while still having the expertise of the nurses and doctors close at hand. It can be a very reassuring experience. This is the time to focus on preparing for discharge. This is a rehearsal for homecoming!

♥

The transfer happened very suddenly. I came to the NICU and they told me he was being transferred that day. I was sad to leave his first home.

There was a huge difference between the units. I was very confident at the first NICU, as there always seemed to be lots of nurses around. But at the next unit, I felt like my baby was not being watched as closely. It made me very nervous. Eventually they explained that our baby was healthier and stronger now and he didn't need all that close monitoring. It would have helped to have known that ahead of time.

The transfer was a big moment for me. It was actually a celebration, kind of like graduation. The new NICU was closer to home, so my life became much easier. And they were way more relaxed. I could pick her up without asking and do most of the care. It wasn't as intense as the other unit . . . I felt more relaxed and gained confidence in the care of my baby. I made up a little card including her likes and dislikes for my baby's bed. It helped the staff get to know her more quickly.

Discharge criteria

Your baby will likely be discharged when healthy and able to feed and grow. Each hospital has its own criteria for safe discharge. The health care team will review your baby's progress in relation to these criteria.

Babies are ready to come home when they:

- maintain normal body temperature in a bassinet (cot);
- feed by mouth, either by breast and/or bottle, safely and effectively;
- have a positive weight-gain pattern;
- are medically stable (no infection, able to maintain oxygen levels);
- do not have an absence of breathing (apnea) or drop in heart rate (bradycardias, or "bradys").

Some "gray areas" may affect discharge timing. For most NICUs, neither a specific weight nor gestational age determine the discharge date. Your baby could go home at 1,800 grams (4 lbs.) or 4,500 grams (10 lbs.). Your baby might be thirty-six weeks' gestation (one month early) or forty-six weeks old (six weeks beyond your due date). Your baby might go home without or with oxygen. Some babies are discharged while still tube feeding. See chapter 3 for our expert advice on caring for babies on oxygen and chapter 4 for advice on tube feeding at home.

Discharge was an unexpectedly difficult experience. We spent months longing for the day we could take our son home, but when it was proposed that he go home, we felt unprepared and anxious. I lacked confidence in my ability to care for him without a team of medical professionals around me 24/7. Due to his medical difficulties, I was also very anxious about not having monitors at home to tell me he was doing okay. We delayed discharge by more than a week to give us more time to room in with him at the hospital, spend time with him off monitors, and take over more of his care with less support from the medical team. That made a big difference for us. We were still anxious, but we felt more confident in our ability to care for him at home.

Plan the trip

It is not possible to predict far in advance exactly when your baby will be ready for discharge. We recommend not asking the health care team for a prediction as your heart will become set on this date. You will be very disappointed if your baby is not ready on that date when you have made big plans, such as arranging for family to travel in. We have seen this happen all too many times.

Without a specific discharge date to count on, parents benefit from some warning about when discharge is nearing. As you will discover, parents need to learn a lot of information and skills before the baby is discharged. A little notice is helpful so that you know when to ramp up your participation in care so that YOU are ready at the same time as your baby.

Oral feeding is a good indicator of readiness for discharge. Once your baby nears 50 percent of total feeds, you should become increasingly involved with your baby's care. This means that your baby is swallowing half of the desired volume and using tube feeding for the remainder. For example, if your baby needs 60 ml (2 oz.) every three hours in NICU, the 50 percent mark would be when your baby feeds 30 ml (1 oz.). Or your baby breastfeeds and needs half a desired feed volume by gavage tube. Becoming more involved when your baby reaches the halfway point will avoid surprise when your baby is really close to discharge. Some babies will sail quickly from 50 percent to full oral and be ready for discharge in a week or two. Some babies, however, will take a long time to get to full oral. In particular, babies who were very premature or medically compromised will need extra time to figure out how to feed well. Be patient.

♥ *During the last couple of weeks in the NICU, I truly started to feel like a mom. My husband dropped me off in the morning and I worked with him all day. I learned that some feeds went well and some didn't. I saw what he was like after feeds. He just couldn't be laid down right away. The nurses helped me figure out what he needed. I learned a lot and was able to troubleshoot feeding problems with the nurses. I became comfortable with all his care.*

Spending long periods of time in the NICU is valuable in teaching your baby to feed and becoming a feeding expert yourself. You will both be ready to go home!

Discharge for twins and triplets

Some families are faced with taking one twin or triplet home when others remain in the NICU. There are pros and cons to taking one home rather than all at the same time. On the pro side, this gives families a chance to adjust to having a baby at home and allows them to get settled before the others are discharged. However, with one baby at home it can be challenging to get back to the NICU to support the other babies.

Here are parent tips about taking home one multiple:

- *Tell the NICU team if you wish to stay at home with the first baby for a couple of days to sort life out.*
- *Ask the team if you may bring the "home baby" when visiting the "NICU baby."*
- *Request a bassinet for your NICU baby's bedside.*
- *Set up a schedule for visiting and balancing life at home.*
- *Ask friends or family for help at home.*
- *Take a day at home occasionally to help you adjust.*
- *Inform the NICU staff of your needs.*

Leaving part of your heart behind

It can be very emotionally difficult to take your baby home when another multiple has died. Conflicting feelings will surface. Parents may feel happy and sad at the same time. You will likely feel a mixture of emotions at memorable moments, for example, when your baby starts to roll or walk, talk, or start school. This will get easier with time but will always remain with you.

How could I feel happy about taking my boy home? I would catch myself smiling or feeling excited and then a wave of intense sadness would flood me as I remembered that my girl will never come home.

Take advantage of professional bereavement support in the hospital, which can help with the grieving process. Before you leave the NICU, ask your nurse or social worker for information about perinatal and infant loss programs in the community and consider joining them.

Some parents have a special memento that keeps their lost multiple's memory alive, such as a special Christmas tree ornament, teddy bear, or wall hanging. You might want to save some photos and mementos (a lock of hair, footprint, or handprint) to share with the surviving siblings when they are older.

We lost the smallest triplet in the NICU. At home, we chose a blue knit heart to represent him in our lives. When we took pictures of the other two boys, we always included that little blue heart. Even years later, we pack the blue heart with us on vacation. He's always a part of us.

I found a foot charm and put it on a necklace. Every so often, I wear that necklace to remember her. I love touching it to remember that she was loved and is missed.

Look for special events in your community to raise awareness for infant loss, for example, some cities hold a "walk to remember" on October 15, and some have a memorial area to plant a tree. Some hospitals have an annual memorial service.

Find someone you can talk to about your feelings. Some parents report that a counselor is the best confidant because your family and friends cannot truly understand your feelings. You don't need to burden them with the mixture of emotions you are experiencing. They may tire of hearing about your pain and joy. Parent groups are often a helpful source of like-minded support. You don't need to go through this alone.

Supplies for the big trip

Gathering your supplies in advance will decrease the stress of discharge and allow you to be present in the NICU to focus on getting to know your baby and the care they'll need at home.

Have the basics on hand:

- ☑ Barrier cream for baby's bum
- ☑ Bottles, nipples, and sterilizing equipment
- ☑ Bouncy chair, swing, front pack, or wrap to carry baby
- ☑ Breast pump
- ☑ Car seat
- ☑ Change mat
- ☑ Clothes
- ☑ Crib or bassinet and required sheets
- ☑ Diaper bag or small backpack
- ☑ Diapers and wipes (unscented, perfume- and chemical-free)
- ☑ Formula
- ☑ Hand sanitizer
- ☑ Normal saline nose drops/nasal aspirator
- ☑ Receiving blankets, sleep sack
- ☑ Soother
- ☑ Thermometer

A bassinet is useful, as you can move it from room to room and it becomes a familiar sleeping surface for your baby. A crib may not fit into your bedroom, so a bassinet is more practical. Do not purchase crib bumper pads or sleep positioners as these increase your baby's risk for sudden infant death syndrome (SIDS).

Ensure the car seat is rear-facing and appropriate for your baby's weight. Do not buy "non-regulated" infant support inserts, such as head rests, pillows, or other comfort items, for use inside the car seat. You must not put anything between your baby and the car seat. Use only manufacturer-recommended products for the car seat.

Don't buy a lot of preemie clothing. Your baby will grow out of these quickly!

A sleep sack is useful in lieu of heavy blankets that may overheat your baby or cover your baby's face.

Before purchasing bottles and sterilizing equipment, ask your nurse about an appropriate bottle/nipple system for your baby. Bottles come in various sizes, shapes, and flow rates. Some nipples are regular (narrow like the NICU nipples) and some are wide. Some are straight and some are "bumpy." Most newborns leaving the NICU need a slow-flow nipple that is regular shape (narrow) and straight (just like the NICU nipple). Take a used NICU nipple to the store to choose a commercial nipple similar in shape.

If purchasing a soother, bring a sample of the soother that your baby is using in the NICU. Ensure the size and shape of the soother are the same. If your baby is bottle fed as well, we recommend the soother and bottle nipple be the same shape and size.

Use formula as recommended by your baby's doctor. This may be a powder that you add to breast milk or might be made with water. The formula might be specialized for your baby's dietary needs. The NICU dietitian or nurse will be a good resource for you. Don't buy formula too soon, as it may change prior to discharge. Special formula can be very expensive. Find out if your health insurance can cover the cost of specialty formula.

Normal saline nose drops and nasal aspirators are helpful to keep your baby's nose clear. There are many different types of nasal aspirators, some are manual (for example, a bulb syringe) and some are battery operated. Ask your baby's NICU nurse to show you how to instill nose drops and use the nasal aspirator.

For breast pumps and supplies, check with your insurance plan, as some insurance companies cover the cost of breast pumps. Ask your nurse or lactation consultant about pump recommendations. Pumps may be manual or electric, single or double. For long-term pumping, consider an electric breast pump with double tubing to save you time. You and your baby may also need a breast shield to support breastfeeding. Check with a lactation consultant to ensure you have the correct size.

For future consideration: you won't need one immediately, but you might want to purchase a stroller that lays flat, as this will be very handy for appointments or walks. Also consider acquiring a bouncy chair, bath tub, change mat, and swing. Consider secondhand equipment as these items are used for a short time. A baby monitor is helpful to allow you to hear and/or see your baby when they are not in the same room. This is not a medical grade monitor or apnea home monitor, which a doctor would order. Very few premature babies need such monitors.

If you have multiples, look into a local multiples club that may have supplies for loan. These clubs may also have annual sales of used baby supplies.

Reduce reliance on monitors

Monitors can be captivating and families come to rely on them. We often see parents sitting by their baby's bedside with their hand on their baby and their eyes directed to the monitor. Parents will also stare at the monitor while babies are feeding.

♥ *It's really hard to not look at the monitor! I stared at that thing for hours. But I knew I had to stop. I was so anxious. I needed to learn to live without wires and numbers, I needed to learn how to read my baby not the screens. My advice to other parents is to turn your chair away from the monitor. Once your baby is stable enough, spend time with your baby OFF monitors. Get used to reading your baby.*

Often it's stressful for parents when the monitor is removed. To gain confidence about being without the monitor, get to know your baby's normal appearance:

- What is your baby's normal skin color?
- What is the normal color of your baby's lips?
- What does your baby's normal breathing look like?
- How fast does your baby normally breathe?

♥ *The nurse took him off the monitor, let me feed him without it, and sat beside me so that we both knew he was safe. It built my confidence tremendously. A couple of weeks before he came home, I was learning what to watch for and what to do.*

The next time you are with your baby in the NICU and your baby's monitor rings, look at your BABY, not the monitor. What do you see? Does your baby look different than they do normally? Is your baby breathing? Look at the color of your baby's face and lips. Is your baby pale or pink? Is your baby active or limp? Most alarms are "false alarms" and you will be reassured to see that your baby is fine and has just pulled off the monitor lead or is kicking actively. What you see and hear is more accurate than a monitor.

You might want to look at taking an infant cardiopulmonary resuscitation (CPR) course. Doing so may increase your confidence in handling emergencies and choking events.

Focus on feeding

The biggest hurdle before hospital discharge is for babies to feed safely and effectively. Heed this mother's advice:

> *This wasn't my first rodeo. I had had a baby three years ago and I thought I knew babies. But this was my first premature baby. I hate to admit it, but I was not ready. I mixed the formula wrong and I didn't feed him enough. He was hungry after feeds and I didn't know why. He lost a lot of weight and had to be readmitted for a week. I wish I had spent more time learning about feeding in the NICU in the first place.*

We strongly encourage you to spend extra time in the NICU to work on feeding. Parents report that this additional work is the most important thing you can do to smooth the transition home.

> *Feeding at home was the number-one stressor. I was so thankful I had spent all that time in the NICU learning from the nurses. Not all feeds are the same and I had to know whether this was okay or not. The nurses gave me tips about how to change from feeding every three hours to following my baby's cues. It was so hard to let go of that schedule.*

To ensure feedings are safe, effective, and pleasurable at home, change to a commercial nipple several days before discharge from the NICU. Made from more durable material than hospital nipples, commercial nipples last for months of use and cleaning, whereas hospital nipples are designed for a single use. A handful of NICU nipples "just in case," does not help your baby in the long-term. Switching to a commercial nipple in advance will avoid the frantic search for the appropriate nipple after your baby has been discharged.

Your baby's bedside nurse can share many feeding tips and strategies. While you are in the NICU, troubleshoot with your baby's nurse about:

- how to clean bottles and nipples;
- how to prepare fortified breast milk or formula (if needed);

- what feeding strategies your baby needs;
- what helps your baby calm down if too upset at the beginning of a feed;
- what to do if your baby falls asleep mid-feed;
- what to do if your baby doesn't take a good feed;
- what to do if your baby wants more;
- what to do if your baby is restless or spilling during a feed;
- what to do if your baby is fussing between feeds;
- what to do if your baby spits up after feeds;
- what to do if your baby throws up an entire feed.

Have a notebook handy to write down the nurse's tips. Once you are home, all the strategies may not be needed for every feed, but you will feel confident that you are prepared for any feeding challenge.

Additional supports for complex health issues

Ask the social worker, nurse, or discharge planner in your NICU about additional supports and services available for you and your baby with complex or multiple health issues. These services differ province to province, state to state, and country to country.

The following may be available:

- Accessible parking permit.
- Parent parking passes for babies with many medical appointments.
- Special needs/disability tax credit.
- Child special needs/disability benefit.
- Health insurance coverage.
- Government programs for support, such as equipment costs, transportation, in-home care, and caregiver relief.

Oxygen at home

If they are medically stable and their parents learn the necessary care, babies may go home on oxygen.

Reasons for sending a baby home with supplemental oxygen include:

- very premature or very low birth weight babies;
- evidence of oxygen desaturation/desat (low oxygen levels) when breathing room air while awake, at rest, or with activity such as feeding;
- long-term stay in the NICU;
- airway problems, tracheostomy, or ventilator (breathing support).

If your baby needs to go home on oxygen, most of the arrangements will be made for you. Exactly how this plays out will depend on your NICU. Some NICUs will contact an oxygen company to arrange to set it up in your home. Some NICUs will ask parents to choose the oxygen company and the NICU will make the rest of the arrangements.

If you are responsible for choosing an oxygen company, consider the following:

- What is the startup fee and monthly fee? What is included in that fee?
- Do they have twenty-four-hour service, and service on holidays?
- What is the company's promised response time if you run out of supplies?
- What are the extra costs, such as for nasal prongs, tubing, tape?
- Does the company recommend humidification of the oxygen?
- Does the company have special cheek tape patches for babies?
- If you are planning a trip with your baby in the next six months, how can the company assist you? For example, are they a national/international company that can provide oxygen tanks at your destination?
- What do other parents recommend?

Whatever system you get at home, don't worry—somebody from the company will be there to make sure you know how to use it. Your instruction in home oxygen use will begin before discharge to give you an opportunity to ask questions and practice using the equipment.

Rooming-in (staying over at the hospital) with your baby and the oxygen equipment is an excellent way to learn. Rooming-in is also a good time to practice a "road trip" as you walk through the hospital with your baby in a stroller and the oxygen equipment. The oxygen company will deliver a small, portable tank to the hospital for travel home. Be sure you know how to confirm that your baby is receiving the correct amount of oxygen.

Oxygen supply companies will share lots of knowledge and help solve issues with equipment. The company will send out a specialist to set up the oxygen equipment in your home and ensure you know how to use the equipment. Some companies periodically send a respiratory technologist to your home to check your baby's oxygen-saturation level. The company should supply an "oxygen in use" sign for your front door.

If your baby needs oxygen at home, don't think of the oxygen as a negative, rather look at it as a facilitator so that you can bring your baby home sooner. While bringing a baby home on oxygen may seem daunting at first, the oxygen will quickly become part of your routine.

> *When they told us our baby would be coming home on oxygen we totally freaked out. We thought we wouldn't be able to handle it. But the hospital staff prepared us so well. By the time we were ready to go home, we were confident in handling the oxygen and our baby. Although the first few weeks were challenging, it quickly became a part of our life.*

See the section "Special Care for Babies on Oxygen at Home" in chapter 3.

Tube feeding at home

Some babies are discharged home before they are fully feeding by themselves.

Reasons a baby may go home on tube feeding include:

- slow oral feeding progress and a long hospital stay;
- baby cannot be fed orally, for example, because of the risk of aspirating liquid into lungs;
- baby has gastrostomy tube;
- parents are willing to take on tube-feeding responsibility.

To take a baby home on tube feeding is a big decision for parents and families. Parents will receive education and training about how to insert gavage tubes, feed by tube, and clean the supplies. You will be able to practice care while your baby is in hospital. Ask lots of questions. Be sure you feel confident about your ability to insert the gavage tube. If your baby will be fed with an electric pump, practice setting the rate with your baby's nurse.

Before leaving hospital, know:

- how to tape the feeding tube in place;
- how to protect your baby's skin and what to do if your baby's skin is irritated by the tape;
- what to do if your baby pulls out the tube;
- where to order supplies;
- who to call if you have questions and whether there's a twenty-four-hour phone number;
- who will give you guidance about advancing feedings;
- if there is special health care coverage for the equipment and supplies.

For more information, see "Tube feeding at home" in chapter 4.

Medications/prescriptions

Fill your baby's prescriptions before you leave the NICU and show the medication to your NICU nurse to ensure that it is the correct dosage. Find out what the prescriptions cost so you are prepared. Practice giving medications in the hospital under the supervision of your baby's nurse. Be sure you know exactly how much and how often to give these medications. Ask your NICU nurse for a few extra syringes for home.

Premature babies often require several medications, such as:

- **Caffeine to reduce the risk of apnea.** Caffeine helps to open up the lung airways and is used to prevent apneic episodes. Usually stopped at four weeks corrected age by your baby's doctor.
- **Vitamins to support life.** In particular, babies need vitamin D. A multivitamin or vitamin E may also be prescribed.
- **Iron to boost red blood cell production.** Most very premature babies need iron for the first six to twelve months of life. Although iron may be upsetting to the stomach, splitting the dose into two and giving it at separate times may help.
- **Folic acid to boost red blood cell production.**
- **Reflux medications to reduce acid production in the stomach.** These also reduce the "acid burn" pain from reflux. Some reflux medications work by increasing the rate at which milk leaves the stomach. Some reflux medications work better when given on an empty stomach, at least thirty minutes before a feed. Ask your pharmacist for instructions.
- **Antibiotics to treat infection.** Antibiotics may upset the stomach and cause loose bowel movements.
- **Thrush medications to treat oral thrush.** These medications are meant to coat the inside of the mouth. These should not be given in your baby's bottle.
- **Diuretics to help the kidneys to remove excess fluid in the body.** These may be given to a baby with chronic lung disease or a heart condition.
- **Blood pressure medications to maintain a normal blood pressure.** Your doctor should monitor your baby's blood pressure while on this medication.
- **Aerosol breathing treatments to help open breathing passages.** The medication is inhaled directly into the lungs.

It is not always easy to give medications to a baby, so it helps to practice in the NICU before discharge. Ask your baby's nurse or pharmacist for directions about when and how to give these medications. If your baby has a lot of medications, ask if any of them can be given at the same time. Ask if these medications should be diluted with breast milk or formula. Find out where to store them, for example in the fridge or in a dark, cool place. Ask for strategies about how to keep track of medications. Tired parents can forget!

Chapter 3 includes more tips for administering medication.

Prepare your home and support system

When you walk out of the NICU with your baby, you want to feel in control of the other necessary parts of life, so you can focus on your baby. Be sure you have everything you and your family will need for three to five days. Make a grocery list and a checklist. Can friends and family help with walking your dog or helping with your older children? Can you use half-day daycare for your toddler? Can your partner take a couple of days off work to help baby settle in at home? What will you eat for the next few days? Fill the fridge! Can a friend or family member buy some groceries for you?

♥ *Double check all you will need for baby, for yourself, and for your house. You do not want to be caught without toilet paper or food and be forced on a trip to the grocery store with a preemie that has just been discharged.*

♥ *Have some healthy food frozen in your freezer. Don't rely on takeout food. We didn't feel very good after a couple of days of pizza. Even a basic casserole would have been a better choice.*

Consider rooming-in

Rooming-in means that you and your partner spend the night or nights in the hospital with your baby. You take over full care and the neonatal team is available upon request. This is a great opportunity for you to really get to know your baby!

You can find out:

- What does your baby's skin feel like with a normal temperature?
- What is your baby's normal tummy appearance?

- How does your baby communicate hunger?
- How loud does your baby cry?
- What does your baby's bowel movement usually look like?
- Does your baby's urine have any smell or color?
- Does your baby hiccup during clothes or diaper changes or while being bathed?
- What calms down your baby?
- How do you swaddle your baby?
- What does your baby do between feeds?
- What sounds does your baby make when sleeping or feeding?

♥ *The best thing we did was stay overnight in the hospital with our babies. This allowed us to take over care with less support from the medical team, but the nurses were just down the hall.*

♥ *We roomed-in for two nights before discharge. Really helpful, but we were exhausted. We hardly slept in that room. It's not like our home. Twin beds, and we were bothered by the hallway noises and room temperature.*

♥ *When we transitioned to home, it was easier than we thought it would be because we already knew about our baby's routine and what to expect. That little bit of comfort was so helpful.*

Most families room-in the night before discharge. You might also room-in a couple of days prior to discharge day and then go home for a good night's sleep before taking your baby home. In either case, parents report that rooming-in gives them the confidence to take their baby home. They also appreciate the opportunity to try full care and ask questions of the neonatal team prior to discharge.

Be prepared for information overload

Expect that a lot of discharge information will be shared prior to discharge. Although NICU staff try to provide this information early and gradually, over time, undoubtedly the information shared just prior to discharge can be overwhelming.

♥ *Before leaving the NICU, I made a list and got the team to answer all my questions. These were about medications, sleeping patterns, when I needed to call the doctor or take baby to the emergency, and about daily concerns like special cleaning routines, using the humidifier, outings, laundry, pets... No question was off the table. I wasn't leaving the hospital without knowing everything possible. I knew we were not going back!*

Ensure you feel comfortable with the following:

- ☑ Feeding, changing, holding
- ☑ Taking temperature
- ☑ Giving medications
- ☑ Storing breast milk
- ☑ Making formula
- ☑ Cleaning bottles and nipples
- ☑ Positioning safely in car seat
- ☑ Giving infant CPR
- ☑ Giving basic first aid
- ☑ Positioning for sleep and SIDS prevention
- ☑ Arranging vaccinations
- ☑ Accessing resources (who to call with questions, for example, a twenty-four-hour telephone advice line)

D-Day

Earlier in this chapter, we stated that your baby's discharge date will likely change.

Discharge dates are set with the best intentions. Leaving the NICU depends on many factors, including your baby's cooperation! Have your home and supplies ready but be prepared for change.

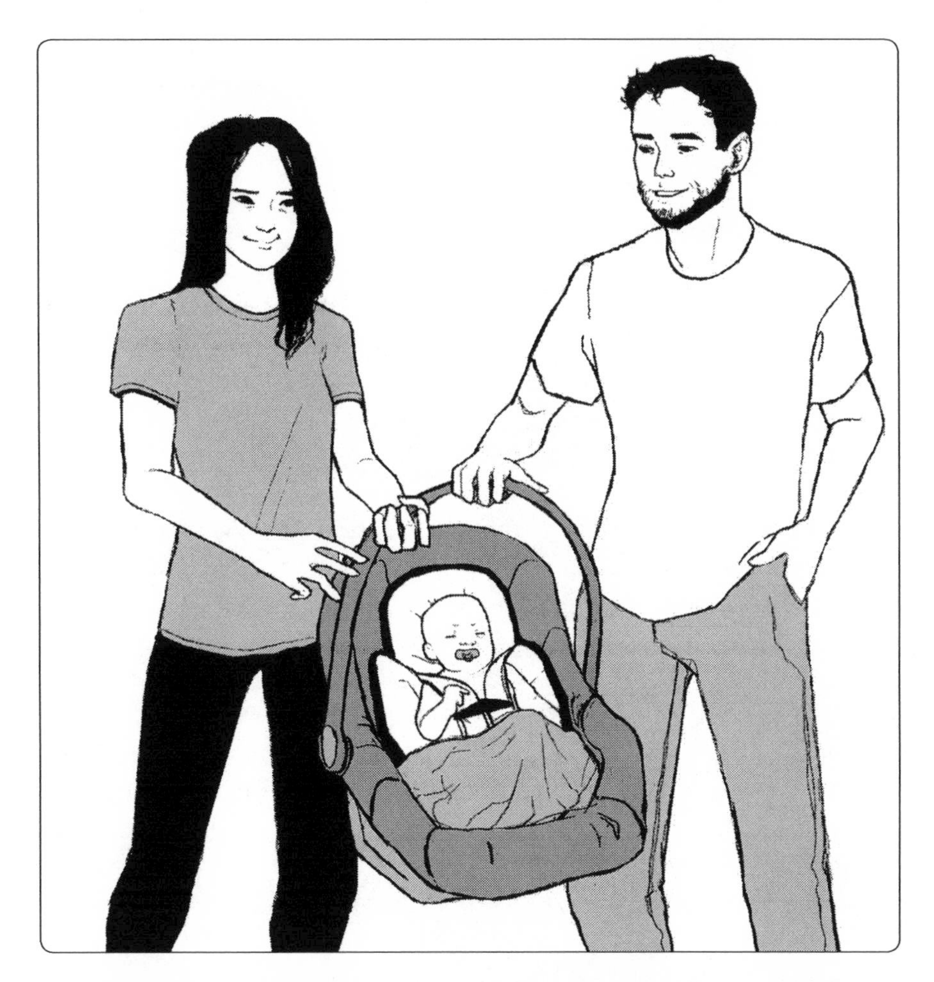

You will thank yourself for being prepared ahead of time for your baby's discharge.

♥ *My mom wanted to come help when our baby came home. She booked her flight for the day of his planned discharge, but a couple of days before that he had a setback and needed to stay longer, so it cost Mom money to change her flight and it was a hassle. We couldn't get a flight on the day we wanted so she couldn't be there for the day he came home. I was sad about that. But, in the end, it was a good thing I had a couple of days before Mom came. It gave my baby and me a chance to figure things out.*

Discharge will happen... eventually. Hang in there! Be ready early, because you might be surprised one day when they announce that your baby's ready TODAY!

At the time of discharge, you will be given:

- discharge instructions about medications;
- a recipe for formula preparation or breast milk fortification as necessary;
- contact information for medical follow-up (for babies who were very premature or were very sick, you may see a lengthy list of future appointments, such as vision, hearing, heart, surgical, neonatal follow-up; get the phone number and address for each clinic);
- a record of the vaccinations given to date.

Ask for information to be written down or take notes. Ask for a medical summary of your baby's NICU stay. This is a helpful reminder and a good resource if you move or change doctors.

All premature babies will have a medical doctor for follow-up. This doctor may be a general practitioner (family doctor or nurse practitioner) or a pediatrician (baby specialist). The doctor assigned to your baby will depend on your baby's health history, ongoing medical needs, and whether a doctor is available in your area or accepting new patients. If your baby is referred to a pediatrician, follow-up may last several months or many years, depending on your baby's needs.

For the remainder of this book, we will use "your baby's doctor" to refer to the general practitioner or pediatrician who is responsible for your baby's general health follow-up.

Post-Departure

When you finally arrive home with your baby, you'll likely wonder how to survive the first few weeks. In our practice, we've seen babies thrive and others struggle at home, and we've seen families excel and others fall apart. The first few weeks home can be rocky.

Below we describe our top tips to ease the transition home, along with offering expert advice from parents.

Follow NICU advice—at first

The transition home is challenging enough for your baby. New sounds, new smells, new bassinet or crib. Keep the rest of your baby's routines as close to the NICU's as possible: use the same breastfeeding and bottle-feeding plans, feeding positions, and bottles. Consistency is important for babies to settle into their new home and routines. Let your baby get used to life at home before you make changes.

Talk to your partner or family about how you want the first few days to flow. Can you take "shifts"? Can someone whom you trust come in during the afternoon to follow your instructions so that you can take a nap? Do you want any company or help? When do you want help to start? Discussing your plans for the first couple of days will help you to relax and enjoy your baby and the wonderful experience of finally being home together. Planning will help you and your partner avoid bickering about little things. Maybe write down your plan and post it for family and friends to see what your goals are.

♥

They told us consistency from NICU to home was important so we made a pact that we were going to follow the NICU way of feeding, burping, and bathing exactly. We even took pictures of the nurse doing demonstrations. We didn't have to correct one another when we got home. We worked like a well-oiled machine. And then Grandma came. She had fed so many children and grandchildren, but there was so much to teach her about preemies.

Once your baby settles in, you can start relaxing the attention on scheduled feeds, precisely timed medications, and exact measurements and weights. Let your baby guide you! Vitamins don't have to be given at exactly eight o'clock every morning. It's okay if you don't record everything your baby drinks today. It's time to get to know your baby and enjoy having them all to yourself.

♥

Feeling empowered to make changes is exhilarating. I can do this by myself! I'm not changing big things, like oxygen, medications, or fortification, but I'm making small changes with feeding and routines, because I can see my baby is ready.

Make one change at a time and assess how each goes. Don't make multiple changes or you won't know what worked and what didn't. If you make a change and it doesn't go well, that doesn't mean it never will. For example, you might increase the bottle volume and your baby throws up. This doesn't mean that your baby will never take more volume. It just means that it didn't work today and you can try again another time.

Set up your home

Keep your home at the same temperature as usual. You don't need to raise the temperature. A good rule of thumb is to dress your baby with one more layer than you are comfortable in. Monitor your baby's temperature. If your baby's temperature is low, see chapter 3 for strategies to warm a baby.

Keep the light and sounds subdued. Your baby is not used to the quiet and dark. Transition from the noisy and bright NICU takes time. See chapter 3 for strategies to help your baby sleep.

> *He just wasn't as calm as in the NICU. He wanted to be held and chill. I think he was just taking in the dog, and the different stuff, the new routines, sounds, and smells. Even the crib—I think it was a struggle because it was not the same bed that he had in NICU.*

Make your home as convenient as possible for managing baby care. A portable bassinet can be moved about your home so your baby has a safe sleeping surface anywhere. If there are two rooms in which you plan to sit frequently with baby, ensure needed supplies are within arms' reach, perhaps in a packed backpack or stocked bassinet. If you have more than one level in your home, supply each with the basics, such as diapers, diaper cream, cloths, clothing, soothers, and a breast shield. You don't want to walk up and down stairs repeatedly. Some families can afford to have a small fridge and bottle warmer near the bedroom to make nighttime feeds easy.

Sleep when your baby sleeps

Sleep deprivation is common after taking a newborn home. Sleep deprivation can be worse when taking a baby home from the NICU because parents might be more anxious and premature babies may give confusing cues and not sleep as well.

> ♥ *Prepare for no sleep. Feeding eight or more times a day, breastfeeding, bottle feeding, pumping, cleaning bottles, sterilizing, changing diapers, and eating. That wiped me out. I was lucky I didn't get sick. I didn't take this advice, but in hindsight I wish I did . . . sleep when the baby sleeps!*
>
> ♥ *I found it tough to sleep because of all the little noises he made. He'd grunt and groan and move about. He didn't sleep well at night so we added a radio and little light. It's hard to sleep through that when you are used to a quiet, dark room. Eventually, I was tired enough that I'd sleep though nearly anything!*

You need sleep. Lack of sleep influences your ability to think and function and affects your health, both physical and mental. If your partner is back at work, that person needs good sleep to be able to function, too. Take turns getting a good block of sleep. Set your priorities. Decide on the really important things to do each day. If you and your baby are fed well, consider that a good day! Take advantage of every opportunity to sleep, even if it's only for half an hour.

Set limits for visitors

Your family and friends will be excited to meet your new family member, just as you will be to show off your baby. But you don't want to expose your baby to germs that will result in a readmission. (See chapter 3 for details on how to reduce the risk of communicable disease.) Premature babies are at a greater risk of rehospitalization in the first year of life, typically for a respiratory illness. Screen your visitors for whether they've been sick in the last few days (sore throats, coughs, runny or congested noses, fever). You can have visitors, but you need to be careful to protect your baby.

Having visitors at your home is a great way to socialize, have "adult conversations," and give you a break from the isolation and hard work of parenting. However, you may choose to restrict visitors for the first few days or weeks. You may limit visitors to close family and friends only. You might choose other parents you met in the NICU as your social network. You might want to kindly request that no young children visit for a while. You might wish to control the length of visits so you don't get too tired. Visiting for four hours means you miss a nap. You might suggest visitors come for coffee or a meal (better yet, bring a meal). When family members want to come for longer periods of times, such as two days or two weeks, consider whether this visit is best to be postponed for a little while. The bottom line is that some visitors will be helpful and some will greatly increase your workload. Set limits on those who are likely to be a burden.

> ♥ *By making friends with other moms in the NICU, I already had a circle of like-minded friends I could talk to and get together with for coffee at one another's houses as a break and for support and adult interaction. We all understood what the other had been through. We were all paranoid about our babies getting sick. We found strength in each other. This really helped to decrease the isolation and loneliness.*

Visitors are potentially a great source of help. Welcome those who will bring a meal or play with your other children while you nap; who won't mind if you lie down for an hour while baby is sleeping; who will fold laundry over coffee.

> ♥ *Never, ever pass up an opportunity to get help. My girlfriend never let a load of clean laundry just sit there. Bless her!*

Don't stress about advice

You will get lots of advice from other people—and only sometimes because you asked for it. Sometimes the advice flows when you really don't want to hear it.

♥ *I love my family but they drove me crazy with all their advice. My baby was twenty-three weeks and had lots of trouble with feeding and reflux. They would say, "You should do this... Don't do that... Try this... Try that..." I told them why their advice wouldn't work and was opposite to the nurse's instructions, because my baby was premature. Many times we had arguments and feelings got hurt, until I lost it one day. My life was already stressful enough. My older sister pulled me aside and told me that I had to pick my battles. She told me to listen quietly and then ignore what I didn't like and keep what I liked. That worked better. Wise sister, eh?*

Most of us can't help giving advice or sharing stories of similar experiences. This is done out of love and not meant to cause stress, but it does for many parents. That older sister was right. Our recommendation is to take advice graciously but with a grain of salt. You decide what is good information. Let go of the rest.

Parents will also receive lots of advice from health care professionals. Sometimes the advice of one specialist contradicts that of another. Perhaps one nurse will tell you to breastfeed only once and another will say to breastfeed for five minutes at every feed. One specialist will tell you to stop a medication and the other one will tell you to increase the dose. Receiving contradictory advice puts parents in an awkward position.

When this happens, tell the practitioner that you have received different information from another specialist. Ensure that they have all the information they need to know about your baby's condition, and let them explain the rationale for their recommendation. Upon hearing their explanation, you can weigh the pros and cons of each strategy. Ultimately you are in control and the expert of your baby. Advocate for your baby and share with the specialists what seems best for your baby. Ask for their advice about how to evaluate whether the plan is working and about the next step. Be up front with your baby's health care specialists. It is better that your health care specialists know the truth than for you to follow a plan without them knowing.

Prioritize and make lists

Prioritize what NEEDS TO BE DONE versus what would be NICE TO DO. Your baby needs to be fed and clean. You need to eat nutritious food. Baby bottles must be cleaned and sterilized. You need to sleep. Housecleaning can be deferred!

A note on the fridge helped me and my family. Whenever we thought of little jobs that needed to be done, we'd post them. The shopping list was there, too. Whenever people came over, they could see all the things to do. My dad was great. He would check the fridge notes and "sign up" for jobs like filling the gas tank, picking up diapers, or putting together the crib. Now if I could just get my in-laws to play the same game!

By writing down the things that need to be done, you won't need to rely on your memory when you're tired and juggling a lot of responsibility. Keep a to-do list and add to it when you think of an item, then relax your mind so that you can "be in the moment" with your baby and not fret about all you want to remember. The item might be cleaning baby bottles, booking an appointment, buying more medication, putting away clean baby clothes, doing yard work, or having the car tuned up. Once it's written down, you know it will be taken care of later. This simple method will reduce your stress and help with household organization. The more organized you are, the smoother your journey will be, especially if you have multiples or other children.

Go with the flow

Depending on your personality type, you might find it hard to be flexible and let go of certain things. Perhaps you are driven to complete everything with perfection or style. You might have been a very clean, organized, well-dressed person before you brought your baby home. And now you are in a whole new situation. The house is messy, you wear sweatpants all the time, and you haven't brushed your hair in days. You might find this stressful!

Some people find it harder than others to be flexible. You and your partner might be experiencing this situation very differently and this can cause stress in your relationship. If your partner is not coping well or acting different reach out for help from your family doctor, counselor, psychiatrist, or psychologist. See chapters 1 and 7 for more strategies on self-care.

Talk about your feelings. Talk about what would make this situation more tolerable. Can you let go of some things, even for a limited time? Consider your priorities and celebrate the great things you are doing. A perfectly clean house is not the priority right now. Think of the stresses of your baby's first few weeks at home as temporary. You can go back to your ideals in the future. The more flexible you are, the less you will stress. Try to go with the flow.

♥ *When I got home, I immediately felt stressed when I saw baby stuff all over and my poor wife with bags under her eyes and wrinkled clothes with spit-up on them. Don't get me wrong, I am the proudest, happiest dad, but this was such a shock to both of us. My wife was having the hardest time. She'd cry about the mess almost every day. I was getting worried about her. I did what I could and told her how beautiful she was and what an amazing job she was doing with our twins. We decided together that the living room would be our baby zone for six months—that it was okay to be crazy messy—just till we could get a handle on everything. Funny thing is, we both learned to relax and enjoy the moment, even in the chaos. Yeah, the living room is full of baby toys now. It's all good.*

Organize appointments

Make a calendar for all of your baby's appointments (there could be lots).

♥ *We missed a couple of appointments and ended up paying a fee for that. Not something we could afford, that's for sure. But there were so many appointments, it was hard to keep them straight. Now I don't leave the clinic before I put the next appointment in my phone. I even have a note app where I record what the doctors tell us. And when the next specialist asks what my baby's plan is, I pull out my phone and give them a report.*

Be sure everyone in the family can see the calendar and be aware of the need to coordinate time and travel for these appointments. Is it possible or necessary for both parents to attend these appointments? Until you feel confident with appointment trips, ensure there are two adults attending, one to drive and one to watch baby in the back seat. If you are heading out to your first appointment with a baby on oxygen you will definitely want help. Later on, you can decide which appointments can be managed by one parent and which ones should be attended by both.

If you are a single parent or if one parent is unable to take time off work, you might consider asking a friend or relative to accompany you and your baby. Community respite programs may be available to assist with medical appointments.

Appointments are disruptive to you and your baby. If your baby has multiple appointments during a week, you might try to consolidate them into one trip. For example, try to schedule appointments in the same vicinity or building on the same day. It might be beneficial to have one heavy day than two days with appointment disruption. Call clinics about the possibility of moving appointments so that they are manageable for you.

Partner in parenting

Just because you are partners or spouses doesn't mean that teamwork will come naturally. Teamwork always works better when individuals talk regularly about plans and consider each person's strengths and limitations. Maybe one partner has returned to work and is away for long hours or at irregular times. Maybe one partner is not feeling well this week and needs extra support. One partner might have more confidence in some parts of baby care. Teamwork will flourish if you take the time to talk about the "game plan" and how to spread out the responsibilities.

♥ *My partner and I have never gone through a crisis like this. Having a premature baby was pure chaos. We didn't know how to function. We bumped along through the NICU like silos. We each did our own thing and never discussed it. A counselor helped us talk about how we wanted to work through this and about how we were better together than working separately.*

At least once or twice a week, check in with your partner to discuss how your game plan is going. Can you divide up the work, including organizing tasks and people and updating extended family and friends? Typically, the stress of transition home from NICU alleviates over time as the volume of appointments eases and your confidence grows. Discuss changes to your game plan and your strategies to balance the responsibilities of baby, home, family, couple, self.

Organize your crew

Caring for a premature baby alone is very hard. If you are a single parent or your partner is away for days and weeks at a time, you carry a lot of responsibility. Don't try to do this alone, as it can be too much for one person.

Figure out who your supports are. Lean on family and friends for help. Let your support people know what they can do to help. Ask them to watch over your other kids, pick up some groceries, make a meal, or babysit while you take a bath or nap. Getting sleep and eating well are real challenges, so if you need extra hands, arrange for them. Asking for help is not a sign of weakness, it's a sign of strength.

If you are a single parent or do not have any supportive people nearby or available, contact your doctor, community nurse, religious leader, or community help line for outreach or volunteer programs. Some communities have free or low-cost volunteers available for childcare or house work. Even two hours of help each week can make a huge difference.

Final Thoughts

The journey home is an adventure. Once you've weathered the NICU, the rocky trip home, the waves of good times and bad, you'll know that you can handle any transition as you create your new normal.

♥ *I promise you that you are on the journey of your life right now. This is not a journey you would have chosen for your baby or family but you will learn things that you wouldn't otherwise know about how strong you are. You have likely met your biggest hero in your perfect miracle. Preemies are incredibly strong and resilient and so are NICU parents. This time will not be easy but you can find magic in it.*

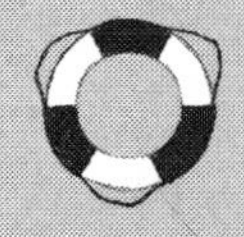

EXPERT TIPS

Here are the key strategies to navigate the journey

- Before NICU discharge, prepare your "life preservers." These are people who are your best sources of support. You'll need help after discharge. It takes more than one adult to care for a recently discharged preemie.
- While your baby is in the NICU, practice all aspects of care and ask all your questions.
- Buy your baby's prescriptions before leaving the NICU and be sure you know how to give them and what they are for.
- Purchase necessary baby supplies in advance of NICU discharge.
- Prepare meals for several days. Ask friends and family for gifts of food. Use prepared meal companies if this is in your budget.
- Stock your fridge with quick, nutritious meals and snacks.
- Delay having visitors and parties until you feel settled.
- Tell your family and friends that you are busy for a while and that you'll be in touch soon.
- Use email/blogs/Facebook/other social media to communicate with loved ones.
- Prioritize you and your baby. Prioritize the must-dos and be willing to let some of the other stuff go. The housework can wait!
- Don't make a lot of changes at first.
- Once you and your baby get acquainted, start to let go of the NICU routines.
- Sleep when the baby sleeps.
- Work together with your partner.
- Use your support systems and tell people what you need.
- If you don't have support systems already, seek them out.
- Enjoy your baby.

KEEPING AFLOAT
Ongoing Health Care for Baby at Home

By the time you arrive at home, your baby will have come a long way from being a small, fragile preemie at birth. However, your baby remains at risk for health concerns. Some babies go home before they reach term and therefore are still premature. Other preemies continue to have fragile lungs or other body systems. Because their immune system is not fully developed, premature babies are more susceptible to illness. Rehospitalization is common in the first year. Extra care is needed to keep your baby healthy and at home.

This chapter contains strategies that are effective in promoting health and preventing illness for premature babies at home. We discuss the most common concerns parents raise, such as how to monitor your baby's health, how to clear your baby's nose, how to reshape your baby's head, how to modify pain, and how to promote safe and longer sleep. You will learn how to minimize exposure to germs, prevent common illnesses and diseases, and what to do if your baby does become sick. If your baby requires oxygen at home, we have lots of special tips for you, too. These tried-and-true methods are an essential part of our clinical practice with parents and are designed to help you keep your baby home.

> *We had her home for hardly a week when it hit me. That urgent need to protect her . . . from crying, from hunger, from other sick people, from injury, from illness . . . even from boredom! I'm always on guard. Is she okay? What does she need? What can I do? In many ways I feel helpless, too. She's our first baby and I admit I don't know anything about babies, let alone premature babies. I need information and advice. I want to be the dad who smoothes the bumps along her life's path.*

This chapter is divided into four major sections: promoting health and preventing illness, special considerations for premature babies, special care for babies who become sick, and special care for babies on oxygen.

Promoting Health and Preventing Illness

In this section we explore strategies to reduce your baby's exposure to germs. You will learn how to monitor your baby's health so that you can tell if your baby is becoming sick. We will also review vaccinations to build your baby's immunity against common illnesses.

Protection from sickness

Every parent's major concern is the possibility that their baby may get sick, or worse, to the point of hospitalization. This is particularly hard on parents of premature babies. You've already spent what likely seemed to be a lifetime in the neonatal intensive care unit. Research shows that premature babies have a 30 to 80 percent risk of being rehospitalized in the first year of life, more than double that of a full-term baby. The most common cause is respiratory infection.

What can a parent do to reduce the risk of respiratory illness? Reduce exposure to smoke and germs. If you can avoid these two contributors, you will go a long way to preventing illness, urgent trips to the doctor or emergency department, and rehospitalization.

Keep your premature baby away from smoke from cigarettes, cigars, or vaping. No one should smoke in the house. Family members should try not to smoke at all, as smoke will cling to their clothes, hair, and breath.

Smoking near your baby irritates their already fragile lungs and increases the risk of sudden infant death syndrome (SIDS, or crib death) and respiratory infections. Smoke paralyzes the cilia in the breathing tubes designed to clear mucus from the airway. When colds or allergies cause more mucus production, the negative effects of smoke on a baby's lungs increase. Smoking can also reduce breast milk production in mothers. Do not expose your baby to smoke.

If anyone in your home smokes, have them:

- smoke outside;
- wash their hands before touching baby;
- change their jacket or shirt before holding baby;
- seek smoking-cessation programs.

Reduce your premature baby's exposure to germs. Infections are a concern for premature babies, but especially for babies with a history of respiratory vulnerability, such as previous respiratory infection or chronic lung disease. If your baby needed oxygen or breathing assistance in the NICU, their lungs need time to heal and grow. A respiratory illness would be a setback.

Airborne germs are spread by coughing, sneezing, laughing, or talking over your baby. Germs can spread up to ten meters (approximately ten yards) and can live on surfaces for hours.

To reduce the spread of airborne germs:

- Avoid contact with people who are sick. If someone is coughing, remove your baby from the area.
- Avoiding kissing or similar close contact with your baby's face and hands when you are unwell.
- Clean surfaces in your home that are touched often, such as countertops and door handles.
- When out for walks or in the presence of other people, consider covering your baby with a light blanket to prevent airborne germs landing on your baby.
- Cover your mouth when you cough or sneeze and then wash your hands.
- If you are sick, try to avoid passing the illness to your baby by good handwashing, reducing direct contact with your baby (you can't totally eliminate contact!), and not coughing or sneezing in your baby's vicinity. Drink lots of fluids, rest, and eat a well-balanced diet. Consider using a face mask, but remember that the protection is reduced once the mask becomes moist from the humidity from your breath.

- If you are well enough to breastfeed or pump, feed your baby breast milk. Sick mothers produce key antibodies in their breast milk.
- Do not let sick older siblings cuddle, kiss baby, or share toys.
- Get help from friends or family who are well.

♥ *I feel like a cop when company arrives. Have you been sick lately? Sore throats? Cough? Runny nose? Fever? No? Okay, then, wash your hands and you can come in.*

♥ *If you are uncomfortable having people come in, just say no. And whoever wants to visit has to follow the rules. In the first months of life, nobody except myself or my husband would feed or bathe the baby. Very few immediate family members would hold her. Handwashing was a must, along with sanitizer and little blankets to cover people's clothes when holding her. After a couple of months we would allow some friends to carry her, but we would ask if they had been sick or in contact with sick people in the past two weeks. Generally everyone was very understanding. And just think of it this way: if someone is really your friend, they will consider your baby's and family's well-being, so handwashing and sanitizing are not a big deal.*

♥ *We had a huge sign saying, "We just got out . . . We don't wanna to go back!!" and placed hand sanitizer all over the house. People got the hint.*

Handwashing is one of the easiest ways to prevent the spread of germs. You likely learned how to wash your hands when your baby was in the NICU. Maintain the correct handwashing technique at home.

Always remember to wash your own hands before handling your baby and require the same of others. Wash your hands after going to the bathroom, handling dirty diapers, or blowing your nose, and, if you are sick, wash your hands thoroughly and regularly.

ACTION PLAN: Handwashing

Try these strategies for handwashing:

- Use liquid soap. A wet, gooey soap bar may not be free of germs. Antibacterial hand soap is not necessary.
- Create friction. This is what removes germs from your hands. Rub all parts of your hands, including between your fingers and under your nails, for at least thirty seconds.
- Use alcohol-based hand sanitizer when you can't wash your hands in a sink. Hand sanitizer may not be effective if you have a gastrointestinal illness or diarrhea.
- Frequently change hand towels.

The common cold

A cold is a viral infection of the nasal passages and throat and can spread into the lungs. A cold can be made worse by dry air (especially in winter months where central heating may be used) or by irritants, such as smoke, dust, or perfumes.

Common cold symptoms may include:

- nasal congestion (your baby may snort or sound "snuffly");
- runny nose;
- increased work of breathing—babies typically breathe through their nose until about four months corrected age; if their nose is plugged, they may not breathe as well and may have an increased breathing rate or show "indrawing" (inward movement of the skin with each breath; seen under the rib cage, between the ribs, or at the top of the breastbone);
- cough;
- sore throat, hoarse voice/cry;
- poor feeds;
- ear infection or ear pain (because the inflammation can also affect the tubes that drain the ears, fluid can collect in the middle ear).

ACTION PLAN: The Common Cold

Try these strategies for managing the common cold at home:

- Provide humidified air to reduce swelling.
- Use comfort measures such as extra cuddles.
- Give smaller and more frequent feeds because appetite may be lower and coughing may aggravate vomiting.
- Monitor how much your baby is drinking and look for signs of dehydration.
- Help your baby's nose stay as clear as possible by following the steps described later in this chapter.
- For babies under three months corrected age with cold symptoms and an abnormal temperature, consult with a health care professional.
- Do not use cold medications without medical advice if your baby is under six months corrected age.

Respiratory syncytial virus (RSV)

Respiratory syncytial virus (RSV) infects the lungs and airways. It is a very common virus in infancy and early childhood, often contracted in crowded areas like daycare centers.

Your baby may have a higher risk of getting very ill from RSV if your baby:

- was born prematurely (before thirty-three weeks of pregnancy) and is less than six months old when the RSV season starts;
- has chronic lung disease or congenital heart disease.

After someone is exposed to RSV, it can take two to eight days before they become sick from the virus and show signs and symptoms of being ill. Peak RSV season is during the winter months or the rainy season in tropical countries. Ask your doctor when the virus is most active in your local area.

In many babies and in most adults, RSV causes mild symptoms and does not require any medical attention.

The symptoms of mild RSV may first present like a cold and can include:

- mild cough;
- nasal congestion;
- runny nose;
- low-grade fever;
- fussiness or irritability.

In most cases, you can take care of your baby at home as long as they are breathing comfortably, their skin does not look blue, and they are drinking and having wet diapers as usual. The infection usually lasts a few days. RSV is a virus and antibiotics will not help, therefore treatment for RSV focuses on relief of symptoms such as fever.

Some babies are at risk for developing a severe form of RSV. This may progress to pneumonia (lung infection) or bronchiolitis (inflammation and mucus buildup in the small breathing airways). These illnesses can be serious and often require hospitalization.

Call for an ambulance if your baby shows signs of respiratory distress:

- **difficult breathing: nasal flaring, indrawing, noisy breathing**
- **rapid breathing (over sixty breaths per minute)**
- **blue lips (cyanosis)**
- **lack of breathing (apnea)**
- **limp, unconscious, unresponsive**

See a doctor within two hours if your baby is unable to keep liquids down or to drink because of congested nostrils, coughing, or feeling unwell; or develops a fever along with cold symptoms.

You can reduce the transmission of RSV by accepting the preventative RSV injection series. The series is available in many countries for high-risk babies, such as babies who were very premature or those with a heart defect. This injection, called palivizumab (pronounced "pal-ee-VEE-zu-mub"), may prevent your baby from catching RSV or reduce the seriousness of illness. Palivizumab is given by needle every three to six weeks during the RSV season and does not interfere with normal infant vaccinations. Reactions are rare; common side effects include temporary clear runny nose, redness at the injection site, and fever. Ask your doctor if your baby qualifies for the palivizumab injection series.

Take baby's temperature

Premature babies have less subcutaneous fat (the fat layer under the skin) and tend to have larger heads (more surface area for heat loss) and be less active than full-term babies. This places them at greater risk of temperature instability. A high or low body temperature can impact your baby's ability to gain weight.

After your baby is first home, you should take your baby's temperature periodically until you have a good sense of your baby's temperature by touching their skin. A digital or mercury thermometer placed in your baby's armpit is recommended. Do not take rectal temperatures. Do not use ear thermometers until your baby is more than six months corrected age as the ear canal is too narrow and will generate an inaccurate temperature. Forehead temperature strips do not accurately reflect body temperature.

A normal armpit temperature is 36.4 to 37.4°C (97.5 to 99.3°F).

ACTION PLAN: Taking Temperature

Try these strategies for taking your baby's temperature:

- Undress the upper body so you can freely access the armpit. You should be able to lift their arm to see where you are placing the thermometer.
- Place the thermometer tip directly into the middle of your baby's armpit.
- Hold the thermometer firmly in the armpit and hold your baby's arm against their body.
- Try holding your baby snugly against your body while the thermometer is reading if your baby does not like having their arm held snugly.
- Know that a digital thermometer will usually register a temperature in less than one minute, depending on the manufacturer.
- Hold a mercury thermometer in place for three minutes.

Observe baby's breathing

A normal breathing rate for newborns is thirty to sixty breaths per minute. Your baby's rate will be faster when crying, upset, or straining. If your baby is breathing fast, help them relax and count the rate of breathing again.

Periodic breathing. A premature baby may have pauses in breathing that last up to ten seconds at a time. This is called "periodic breathing" and is common in premature babies. Even healthy, full-term babies occasionally have periodic breathing, especially when the baby is sleeping deeply. Periodic breathing is not the same as apnea (when breathing stops for at least twenty seconds and baby is limp, blue or pale, and heart rate is low). When a baby has periodic breathing, their color remains pink and they do not go limp. After periodic breathing pauses, your baby may breathe rapidly and then the breathing rate relaxes. A baby with periodic breathing will always resume normal breathing on their own. No stimulation is needed. Although it can be alarming to parents, periodic breathing is a harmless condition and goes away as babies get older.

Indrawing. Most premature babies have mild indrawing when they breathe. This inward movement of the skin during breathing may appear under the rib cage, between the ribs, or above the rib cage. You may remember seeing this when your baby was in the NICU. Indrawing is common in very premature babies or low birth weight babies. Once babies become healthy, older, and heavier (and therefore have more subcutaneous fat), respiratory indrawing becomes milder or goes away. Typically, by the time premature babies are discharged, only mild indrawing remains, primarily slight indrawing of the skin under the ribs. You will learn the normal amount of indrawing for your baby. If your baby's indrawing increases, or if your baby ever has trouble breathing, you should urgently seek medical attention.

Clear baby's stuffed-up nose

Premature babies often make a noisy or squeaky sound from their nose. Their nose passageway is very narrow and can make sounds with secretions. The noise can become worse if your baby's nose is congested. Keeping your baby's nose clear will decrease this sound and make breathing easier. As your baby grows, this sound will disappear.

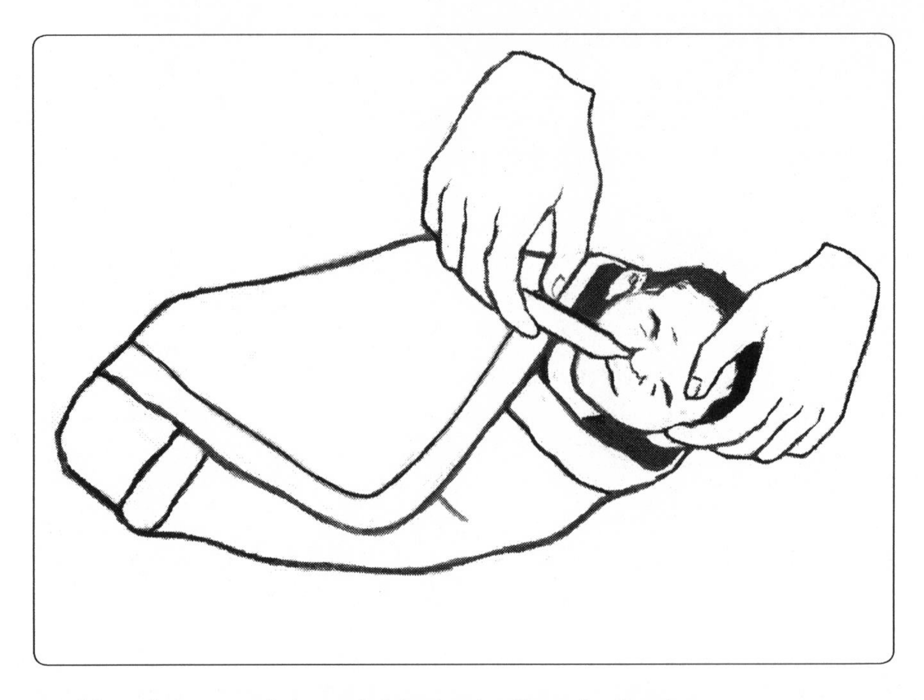

Swaddle and place your baby on their back to instill nasal saline drops.

Moisten your baby's nasal passages with saline drops. You can purchase these from a drugstore or make them at home (dissolve ¼ tsp salt in 125 ml [½ cup] warm water). Lay your baby on their back, as shown in the illustration above. Put one or two saline drops into each nostril. Saline drops may be enough to keep your baby's nostrils moist and clear. A sneeze is the most effective way to clear the nose. When your baby sneezes, look for secretions to wipe away. If your baby is sneezing frequently, use saline drops more often so each sneeze can be effective. The safe storage time for homemade saline drops is unknown so replace periodically. Do not use if the liquid is cloudy.

Use a humidifier or cool-mist humidifier near your baby's crib. Water vapor can help moisten and loosen the mucus inside your baby's nose. Clean out and refill the vaporizer every day. Follow manufacturer directions for cleaning the humidifier. You can also bring your baby into a bathroom steamed up by the shower.

ACTION PLAN: Stuffy Nose

Try these strategies for clearing a stuffy nose:

- Place one to two saline drops into each nostril.
- Use a rolled tissue to wick out secretions from each nostril.
- If you hear or see secretions from the nose, a nasal bulb syringe or an aspirator may be used to remove secretions.
- Don't use nasal bulbs or aspirators unless you can see or hear secretions.
- Over-suctioning can be irritating and cause more secretions.

Vaccinations

Vaccination guidelines vary around the world. In some countries, vaccinations are optional and the focus is on educating parents on the benefits of immunizing their babies and children. There are more than fifteen countries where vaccinations are not mandatory. Other countries offer financial incentives for vaccinating or have made them mandatory to ensure high coverage rates. Several countries with mandatory vaccination policies are challenged to enforce them. The World Health Organization (WHO) is working hard to promote global vaccination coverage for babies: a challenge in developing countries.

Many things for premature babies are based on corrected age, but vaccinations are not. Most countries vaccinate preemies based on their chronologic age (age from birth). So, at six to eight weeks, you will be faced with the decision to vaccinate your premature baby. This can sometimes be a difficult choice, especially if your preemie is still in hospital. Parents may think that their preemie is too fragile to be vaccinated because of small size, gestational age, health problems, and an abundance of pain-causing procedures.

But based on the guidelines for vaccinations and recommendations by pediatricians around the world, premature babies should be given the routinely recommended infant vaccinations. They should receive every vaccination on the standard schedule. Vaccination is the best way to protect your baby from many dangerous diseases, such as diphtheria, tetanus, pertussis (whooping cough), and polio. In some countries, the flu vaccine is recommended for babies once they are six months old.

Here are the top three reasons to vaccinate your premature baby:

1. Preventable illness is more common and severe in preemies.
2. Vaccines work, even in very small preemies.
3. Vaccines are safe for preemies.

Countries make decisions about vaccination recommendations based on a number of factors. Countries must consider the burden of the disease in their region, both in terms of mortality (deaths), overall suffering and disability (how many people get the disease, how severe is it, and its lasting effects), and the cost of that burden compared with the cost of the vaccine. They also consider the effectiveness of the vaccine and its safety profile, including possible side effects. They may also account for what they expect the uptake of a vaccine to be—a vaccine that's recommended but which few people actually get may end up being less cost-effective as a result.

Vaccines are recommended by the WHO for the following diseases:

diphtheria
haemophilus influenzae type b (Hib)
hepatitis B
measles
meningococcal disease (meningitis)
mumps
pertussis (whooping cough)
pneumococcal
polio
rotavirus
rubella
seasonal influenza (flu)
tetanus

For links to vaccination resources, visit our website at www.preemiecare.ca.

There are several common questions that parents ask about vaccinating their premature baby.

Are vaccines safe for premature babies? All of the vaccines available are safe when given to premature or low birth weight babies. Side effects associated with the vaccines are similar in both full-term and preterm babies, with one exception. Very premature babies who are still in the NICU for their first immunizations at approximately two months chronologic age have an increased risk of apnea and desaturations for two days after their shots, especially if they have chronic lung disease (or bronchopulmonary dysplasia [BPD]) or are still on respiratory support. For this reason, very premature babies should be observed in the NICU for at least forty-eight hours after their vaccines. If your baby is still in hospital and is very sick, the NICU may wait until your baby is more stable for the vaccines.

Why can't we wait until our baby is bigger? Premature babies can get a lot sicker than full-term babies if they get the diseases that the shots prevent (especially pertussis/whooping cough). We need to make sure that premature babies get full protection as soon as possible.

What are the risks of not vaccinating or not vaccinating on time? The diseases prevented by infant and childhood vaccines are serious and even deadly. Measles can spread to the brain, causing brain damage and death. There is no treatment and no cure for measles, polio, and tetanus. The only way to protect your child is through vaccination.

Does my premature baby need to get a full dose of the vaccines? Yes. Half or split doses don't work as well. Even small premature babies need the full dose for full protection.

How can I minimize the pain? Ten percent of parents decide not to vaccinate based on the pain their baby will experience. Please see the section below on minimizing the pain of vaccinations as well as our videos on www.preemiecare.ca.

> **Although vaccination is a personal choice, we strongly recommend that you keep vaccinations current for you and your children. *Please* keep in mind that vaccinations not only protect you, but also the most vulnerable: your preemie.**

Buffer baby's pain

It is distressing for parents to watch their baby experience pain. The majority of parents report wishing they could participate in managing their baby's pain.

> *I knew she needed those needles, but I felt so helpless watching her. It killed me to see her pain. My eyes filled with tears. I just hugged her close and told her, "Mommy loves you, Mommy loves you," over and over again.*

The instinct to provide physical presence and reassurance is the most beneficial action a parent can take when their baby (or child) experiences pain.

Babies do feel pain. Every baby's reaction is unique. Babies commonly show their pain in a few ways:

- They initially hold their breath and turn deep red/pink/purple after the shock of the pain. The color returns to normal when deep breaths are taken.
- They wince, grimace, close eyes tightly, and open eyes wide.
- They stiffen their body and try to pull or push away.
- They scream, cry, or whimper.
- Their breathing rate and effort increases.

Yes, it's hard for parents to watch this. You can't take away the pain, but there are many actions you can take to lessen your baby's pain response to a single painful event such as vaccinations, needles, blood tests, eye examinations, the insertion of feeding tubes, and the insertion of intravenous lines.

ACTION PLAN: Painful Events

Try these strategies BEFORE baby's painful event:

- Be calm. Breathe deeply through your nose and exhale slowly during the test. Look away if you need to. If you are stressed, your baby will sense this. If you are calm, you will be a calming force for your baby.
- Breastfeed during the event. Start a few minutes beforehand.
- Give skin-to-skin cuddles; hold your baby securely; wrap your baby snugly in blanket.
- Let your baby suck on a soother or your finger so that natural endorphins are released.
- Distract baby with toys, music, your voice.
- Dab the inside of baby's cheek or inner lip with oral sucrose.

Try these strategies DURING and AFTER the painful event:

- Cuddle your baby to help them feel secure.
- Give baby extra attention and comforting for several hours.
- Distract baby with toys, music, your voice.

- Rock your baby gently.
- Breastfeed or bottle feed for comfort. Your baby may feel comforted by small, frequent feeds for several hours.
- Give baby a soothing bath.
- Avoid touching the area. For example, change your baby's diaper carefully to avoid pressing on the vaccination or heel poke sites.

Oral sucrose is a safe, effective method for reducing short-term pain from a single event such as vaccinations. The sweet taste distracts your baby and stimulates an endorphin release that eases the perception of pain. This analgesic effect starts within seconds and lasts for five to ten minutes. Oral sucrose is most effective for babies and has been reported to be beneficial for infants up to eighteen months old. Oral sucrose is not appropriate for long-term pain.

Oral sucrose may be purchased, or you can make your own:
2 tsp water + 1 tsp white sugar
For babies under four months corrected age, this water should be boiled for two minutes before adding the sugar

Approximately two minutes before the painful event, give 0.2 to 1 ml oral sucrose on the inside of your baby's cheek or inner lip. You may also dip a soother in this solution. You may repeat oral sucrose once or twice if the procedure is delayed. Throw the remaining solution away. Do not store it.

Analgesics and topical anesthetic creams or patches are usually not necessary for short-term single painful experiences. Topical creams or patches are useful if your baby is having an intravenous line inserted or a minor surgical procedure. Unless indicated by your baby's doctor, analgesics and anesthetic patches should not be given before a vaccination or blood test.

If your baby's pain persists despite the above post-event care strategies, consult with your health care provider about the correct dose of acetaminophen/paracetamol for your baby. Give the dose according to your baby's corrected age or current weight. Do not give aspirin or ibuprofen if your baby is under six months corrected age, unless recommended by your doctor.

Routine appointments

You and your newly discharged premature baby may be very busy with appointments in the first two months at home. Your baby's degree of prematurity, birth weight, and health issues will determine the type and frequency of appointments. There are certain routine medical follow-up recommendations.

General health, growth, and development. Some premature babies will be followed by a general practitioner (family doctor or nurse practitioner). Very premature babies are often referred to a pediatrician (baby specialist). The NICU will typically set the first appointment for you or advise you to arrange an appointment within two weeks of NICU discharge. The frequency of these appointments will be related to how well your baby is doing.

Vision. To ensure the blood vessels in the eyes are growing properly. Abnormal blood vessel growth may be called "retinopathy of prematurity" (ROP). The eye doctor will follow your baby closely until the eyes are fully vascularized and ROP has receded.

Hearing. Some maternal illnesses during pregnancy (for example, German measles, herpes); prematurity; newborn illnesses (such as jaundice, infection, meningitis, seizures); long-term ventilation; and newborn medications (for example, gentamicin, tobramycin) increase the risk of hearing loss. Premature babies may have a hearing check while in the NICU or shortly after discharge. Your baby's test results will be a "pass" or "referral." A "referral" result commonly means that one ear or both contains fluid and the test will be repeated in the future.

Oxygen clinic or team. Babies on home oxygen will require specialized follow-up.

Nephrologist (kidney specialist). Babies with nephrocalcinosis (calcium deposits in the kidneys) or blood pressure issues will require specialized follow-up.

Cardiologist (heart specialist). Babies with heart defects or heart problems will require specialized follow-up.

Long-term follow-up. Very premature babies may be referred to a clinic for special follow-up. These clinics often include a variety of professionals such as occupational therapists, physiotherapists, dietitians, social workers, psychologists, and speech therapists.

Here are parent tips about doctor appointments:

- *Take extra supplies for baby. You never know when you'll need to change their clothes.*
- *Pack items for yourself—snacks and something to drink—which can help you function well and keep your wits about you during complex appointments.*
- *For babies with reflux, bring extra blankets, wet facecloths in a baggy, and a change of shirt for yourself.*
- *If you are bottle feeding, pack extra feeds for baby.*
- *Don't forget the breast shield if your baby needs one for breastfeeding.*
- *Bring cool bottled breast milk or formula in an insulated bag with a cold pack.*
- *If you want to prepare formula/fortified breast milk at the appointment, put sterilized water/breast milk in a clean baby bottle. Into a separate small container, place the right amount of powdered formula. When ready to feed, add the pre-measured formula to the bottle, shake, and heat.*
- *Bring a thermos of hot water to heat up bottles.*
- *Avoid the exposure to germs on public transit. If you don't drive, ask friends, family, or neighbors to drive you.*
- *Try to combine more than one appointment on a single day.*
- *If you have a lot of appointments at the same place, look into weekly or monthly parking rates.*
- *Park nearby at a free spot and use a stroller for the walk in.*
- *Look into accessible/handicapped parking criteria, for example, a baby on oxygen may qualify.*
- *If you have a lot of appointments, ask a social worker whether help with transportation is available.*
- *If your baby has complex health issues, write your travel and parking expenses on a calendar and keep receipts. Your baby may qualify for disability expenses and some coverage may be backdated.*
- *Don't forget to buckle your baby into the car seat.*
- *Remove your baby from the car seat after you get to the appointment so that they can breathe properly and not be squished. Use a front pack or a stroller when you arrive.*
- *Be kind to your back and get a stroller. It takes time to set up and take down, but it's so much more relaxing to have storage areas and to be able to put your baby in it sometimes, especially during long appointments.*
- *Babies and parents are fussy after long appointments. Everyone needs extra TLC when you get home!*

Special Considerations for Preemies

Now that you are home with your baby at last, you may be wondering what other things you can do to promote health. In this section, you will learn to promote safe sleep and a round head. As well, you will learn about the benefits of massage and simple techniques that anyone can do. We offer advice on giving medications, when to stop sterilizing bottles, and what drooling and teething mean for premature babies.

Sleep patterns

Babies have periods of active (light) sleep and quiet (deep) sleep. During a long sleep, you will notice that your baby cycles several times between quiet and active sleep. The time from one active sleep period to the next is called a sleep cycle. A full sleep cycle for a premature baby is about thirty to forty minutes. When your baby reaches full term, one full sleep cycle will last about fifty to ninety minutes.

During active, or light, sleep:

- your baby may twitch, squirm, toss a bit, make little grunting noises, or make facial expressions or yawn;
- you may notice your baby's eyelids fluttering and eyes moving under closed eyelids;
- your baby's breathing is irregular;
- your baby will be easily woken by noise or activity in the room.

During quiet, or deep, sleep:

- your baby will sleep peacefully, breathing more regularly and slower than when awake;
- your baby will not actively move, although you might see or hear sucking noises;
- your baby will have a hard time waking up and will want to go back to sleep;
- your baby's body resting, healing, and growing (growth hormone is secreted);
- discomfort or pain will shorten the sleep.

♥

While she was sleeping, she sometimes lay there quietly and then, ten minutes later, she'd be wiggling, making noise, and opening and closing her eyes. She'd make so much noise that she'd wake me up. Not crying, really, just little grunts. I thought she was hungry, but she wouldn't take much. I was worried there was something wrong.

Premature babies spend more time in active sleep. In general, fifteen to twenty minutes of a sleep cycle is spent in quiet sleep and the rest is active sleep. Once your baby is between term and two months corrected age, periods of quiet and active sleep will be closer to equal. As your baby ages, more time will be spent in quiet sleep. Close to two months corrected age, your baby may start sleeping four or more consecutive hours at night.

One big difference between my babies is how they slept. My first baby was full term and just ate and slept. My second baby was premature and didn't sleep as well. She moved about in her sleep and made noises like a little baby goat. When she opened her eyes and squirmed, I couldn't tell if she was waking up or just in light sleep. Eventually she slept better, but that was two or three months after leaving the NICU.

Typical sleep duration

Corrected age	Sleep duration	Awake duration	Total sleep/day
0–2 months	2–4 hours	1–2 hours	16–18 hours
2–4 months	3–4 hours	1–2½ hours	14–16 hours
4–6 months	• begins sleeping longer at night (4–8 hours) • takes little short naps (20 minutes to 2 hours) during day	2–3 hours	12–14 hours
6–12 months	• develops longer night sleep • takes 3, and eventually 2, short naps during day	2–4 hours	10–14 hours

Sleep patterns are unique to each baby. In general, some premature babies do not sleep as long or as deeply as full-term babies. Some babies are long sleepers and others are not. If you are worried about your baby's sleep, write down sleep and wake times for a week and discuss them with your baby's doctor.

Promote baby's sleep (and yours)

Sleeping can be particularly challenging after discharge from the NICU. A lot of babies do not like the dark and the silence at night because they are used to being in the NICU, where there is no "night." They are used to sleeping through noise and activity going on around them. The first few nights and weeks at home can be tough. They may happily sleep all day while everyone is talking or making noise, and then might be wide awake all night. Most newborns will start sleeping better at night by the time they are one month corrected age or home for at least a month.

> *My baby always slept well in her cot in the family room. My three-year-old played nearby, the TV was blaring, lights were on. But the nights were horrible. Both of us became sleep deprived before I realized the family room was like the NICU. Noisy and busy. She slept well there but didn't know how to sleep in the quiet and dark. I couldn't let her sleep in the family room any more. I found a quiet, dark place for daytime naps and that helped a lot.*

ACTION PLAN: Sleep

Try these strategies to promote sleep:

- Before trying to help your baby sleep, be sure there is not a physical reason that your baby cannot sleep, such as being hungry; overfed (has a sore tummy); in a wet or dirty diaper; too warm or too cold; sick; overstimulated (too much activity before sleep time); in discomfort from gas, reflux, or uncomfortable position; in pain.
- Use a consistent location for sleep. Help your baby learn to sleep in their bassinet or crib during the day and night.
- Play soft background noise, such as the sound of a fan or soft music; use a sound machine; or download a white noise app on your phone.
- Use a night light or low-intensity lamp.
- Do not use pillows or heavy quilts.

- Swaddle or bundle your baby. Some babies sleep better when swaddled. The diamond full-body swaddle is the most common (see illustration below). Visit our website at www.preemiecare.ca for links for additional swaddling techniques.
- Use an infant sleep sack correctly sized for your baby's weight. Baby's face should be clear, and enough room should be left for the legs to move.
- Take baby to a quiet area before sleep time. The room should be calming. Speak quietly. Avoid stimulating play or noise before bedtime.
- Notice how your baby responds to stillness versus rocking. Rocking may be too stimulating or gentle rocking may help your baby to relax. Use stillness or rocking to lull your baby.
- Hold baby against your chest while standing and walking or rocking a little. A common parent finding is that the minute you sit down, they wake up!
- Give baby a soother or pacifier. Eventually your baby's need to suck will decrease and the soother will no longer be desired.
- Massage or bathe baby.
- Be patient. There will be a period of adjustment as your baby transitions to the routine of day and night. This may take several weeks.
- Avoid holding your baby for hours between feeds, even though your baby will tend to sleep longer when held. Help your baby get used to their consistent sleeping place.
- Stop using white noise and light once your baby sleeps better at night.
- Avoid waking a baby from deep sleep. Sleep disruption can affect growth and development. If possible, wait until your baby is in a light sleep state, drowsy, semi-alert, or awake.
- Around two to three months corrected age, place your baby in their bassinet or crib when they are relaxed and drowsy but before they are fully asleep. Older babies should fall asleep and awaken in the same location. Help your baby feel secure with bundling or leaving your hands on your baby's body while they relax. Slowly stroke your baby's head. Speak or sing softly.

- Around three to four months corrected age, start a bedtime routine, such as a bath, sitting in certain chair or room, reading, singing, rocking in dark room, saying good night. Keep night bedtime at the same time daily. A consistent pattern helps your baby learn when it's sleep time.
- Around four to six months corrected age, ALWAYS place your baby in the crib before fully asleep. This starts teaching babies to fall asleep by themselves. Avoid eye contact and stimulating conversation or play. Keep bedtime routines.
- Expect that near six months corrected age (or earlier if you are lucky), your baby will be ready to sleep through the night. Older babies will start to learn how to help themselves fall asleep with self-soothing behaviors such as sucking on their fingers or wiggling to get comfortable. They might fuss a little. Babies over six months corrected age do not need to be picked up right away when they fuss. Simply your presence, touch, and voice help them feel secure enough to drift off to sleep.

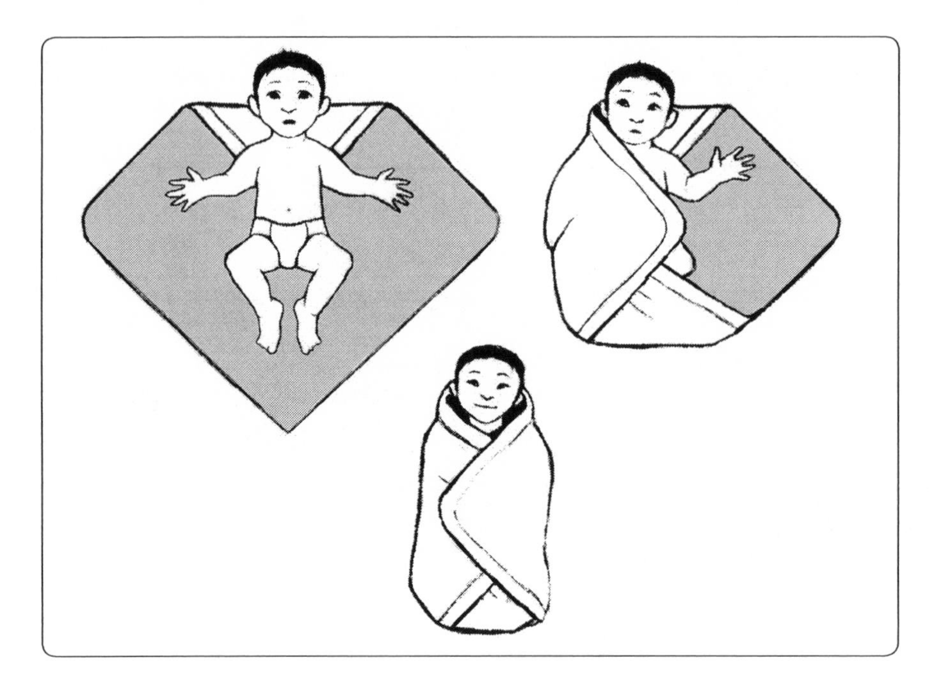

Some babies settle well in this common diamond full-body swaddle. Some babies like their hands out so like to be swaddled from the chest down.

Do not get stressed about your baby's sleep. Don't compare your baby with other babies. With your help, your baby will figure out how to sleep at night and how to sleep longer.

Create a safe sleep environment

In the NICU you may have seen your baby placed on their tummy to sleep. This is safe to do in the hospital as they are closely monitored. Babies are transitioned to sleeping on their backs before going home. At home, all babies, including preemies, should be put on their backs to go to sleep. In fact, it's vital for preemies to sleep on their backs because they are at a slightly higher risk for sudden infant death syndrome (SIDS). Since the start of the "Back to Sleep" program, which recommends that all babies be placed on their backs for sleep, the incidence of SIDS has dropped dramatically.

For the first six months, the safest place for babies to sleep is on their back in a crib or bassinet in your room. If you can't fit the crib in your room, use a bassinet. Having your baby in the same room means that you will be able to hear them when they cry softly. Parents often worry about their baby's sleep and having the baby in the same room means you can keep a close eye on them.

Some parents wonder about bed sharing, which means sleeping on the same surface as their baby. Adult beds are not designed with baby safety in mind. Your bed is not a safe place for your baby to sleep.

Adult beds increase the risk of SIDS or suffocation in the following ways:

- A baby becomes trapped in a space between the mattress and the wall, or between the mattress and the bed frame.
- A baby falls off the bed.
- An adult or an older child rolls over and suffocates a baby.
- Soft bedding, such as comforters or duvets, cover a baby's head and cause overheating. Babies who have their heads covered during sleep are at increased risk of SIDS.
- Co-sleeper products (baby beds that attach to adult beds) are not recommended by many health and safety organizations. They are not supported by Health Canada.

The safest place for your baby is in their own sleeping space, such as a crib or bassinet.

ACTION PLAN: SIDS

Use these strategies to reduce the risk of SIDS:

- For the first year of life, place your baby on their back at nighttime and for naps. Do not use sleep positioners or rolled-up blankets to keep your baby in one position, as this raises the risk of choking and suffocation.
- Use a firm, flat surface for sleep. Waterbeds, travel beds, air mattresses, pillows, couches/sofas, or soft materials are not safe sleep surfaces for babies. Babies can turn onto their side or stomach and bury their face in these soft materials and not get enough air to breathe.
- Do not use car seats or baby carriers for your baby's sleep. If you return home from an outing with your baby asleep in the car seat, take them out and put them in their crib or bassinet.
- Keep soft materials out of your baby's sleep environment. Do not use quilts, comforters, bumper pads, stuffed animals, pillows, or other pillow-like items. Do not make nests like the ones used in the NICU. You want your baby to be free to move and not be stuck in one position.
- Check your baby's temperature to ensure they are properly dressed for sleep. Overheating increases your baby's risk for SIDS. If the room is warm, dress your baby in a one-piece sleeper and swaddle in a light blanket. If the room is cool, add an undershirt. The house temperature should be at whatever is comfortable for you and your baby requires one extra layer. If the tummy and neck are hot and sweaty, remove a layer.
- Keep your baby away from cigarette smoke. Babies whose mothers smoked while pregnant, and babies who are exposed to smoke after birth, are at increased risk of SIDS. Choose non-smoking caregivers for your baby.
- Ensure your baby's crib or bassinet meets the most current safety standards.
- Always place your baby on a flat mattress, which is the safest angle. Tilting the crib mattress raises the risk that your baby may roll to the bottom and be pinned and suffocated. If your doctor advises you to elevate the head of your baby's sleeping areas, get the proper instructions from your doctor.
- Don't fall asleep in an armchair or on a sofa with your baby.

- Don't leave baby sleeping in a playpen for unsupervised sleep. This is not safe. Babies have died as a result of a playpen collapsing or from getting trapped between a playpen and other items when left alone.
- When your baby can roll over on their own (at approximately five to six months corrected age), you don't need to return them to their back.

Head shape and plagiocephaly

A baby's skull is very soft, and the skull bones can be affected by pressure. Babies also have weak neck muscles and usually turn their heads to one side when placed on their back. Because of this, your baby's skull may flatten. The medical term for this is "positional plagiocephaly." Plagiocephaly is characterized by a flattening of one side of the skull.

The best way to see if your baby has a flat spot is by looking from above at the top of their head and assessing if it is symmetrical. Compare your baby's head with the following head shapes.

Head shape A below shows how your baby's head should look. Notice how the ears are opposite to each other. A perfect triangle is formed between your baby's nose and each ear.

Head shape B is symmetrical, but the head is very narrow. This is from lying on the ears too long and not lying on the back of the head. This is called scaphocephaly.

Head shape C shows an asymmetric head shape with the right ear is displaced forward. This baby has been lying on the right side of the head, which has flattened the head behind the ear and pushed the ear and right side of the forehead forward. Right-side flattening is common following long NICU stays.

Head shape D shows that the back of this baby's head is flat. We have often seen this caused by too much time spent with head in midline position, often in a baby bouncy chair or swing. The incidence of flattening at the back of the head (called "brachycephaly," the most common form of plagiocephaly) has increased dramatically since the beginning of the "Back to Sleep" program as part of the prevention of SIDS. Head-flattening may have started in the NICU or may develop at home. It is also more common in premature babies and multiples.

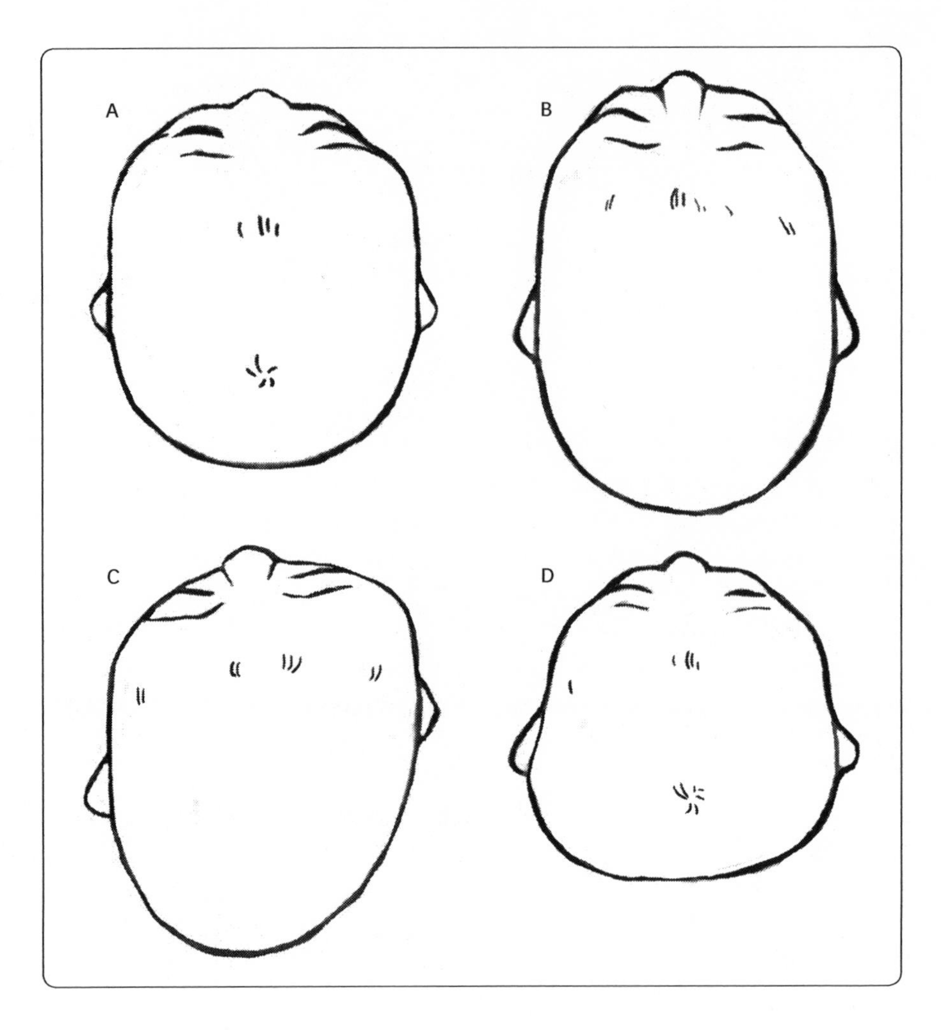

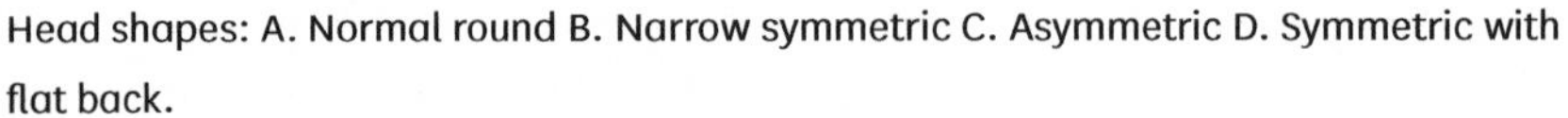
Head shapes: A. Normal round B. Narrow symmetric C. Asymmetric D. Symmetric with flat back.

Most flat or asymmetric head shapes can be prevented, but not always. If your baby's head is nicely round now, be sure they continue to look in directions (right, left, and midline) equally. Watch if your baby shows a preference in turning their head to one side and if they do, or if they have a flat head shape, act now. A baby's head is soft and moldable until three to four months corrected age. The sooner you act, the quicker the head will reshape. If you don't act, the head shape will become permanent after four months corrected age.

ACTION PLAN: Plagiocephaly

Try these strategies to avoid plagiocephaly:

- Alternate your baby's position every day, placing your baby's head toward the head of the crib one day and toward the foot the next. Babies will often look away from the wall to the center of the room or the door, where you and the action are.
- Alternate at which end of the change table you place your baby's head while changing.
- If your baby prefers one side, gently turn their head to the other side. Alternate where you place toys on the crib, stroller, swing, or baby seat.
- If you use an overhead mobile, change the position so that your baby is not looking up all the time.
- Do not place rolls or barriers in your baby's sleeping area as these could increase the risk of choking or SIDS.
- Use rolls to prevent your baby from lying on their ears ONLY when you are present to watch. Rolls can also be placed beside your baby's head in a bouncy chair or swing, provided that you are supervising. If you are not watching closely, do not use any rolls.
- Alternate the hip or arm with which you carry your baby.
- Alternate the side from which you feed your baby.
- Switch your baby's position frequently. Do not let your baby lie or sleep for long periods in a bouncy chair or swing.
- Give your baby supervised tummy time for ten to fifteen minutes and at least three times a day. This means you set your baby down to play on their tummy. Start with one to two minutes at a time and gradually increase the time as your baby tolerates it. Tummy time will help prevent a flat spot on the head and will strengthen their neck and shoulders. (See chapter 6 for more on tummy time.)
- Place your baby on the floor for playtime and encourage your baby to look right, left, and midline.

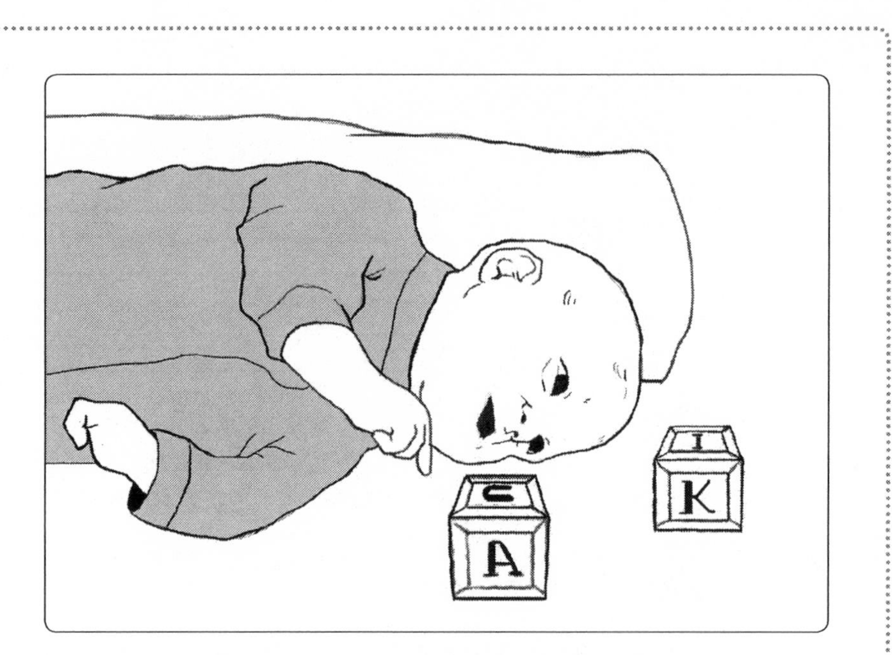

Try therapeutic positioning to correct your baby's asymmetric head shape.

- If your baby has flattening on one side of their head, lay your baby on the other side on a blanket on the floor. See therapeutic positioning to aid head shape as shown in the illustration above. For the best results, use a very thin blanket on a hard floor, rather than a thick blanket or on carpet. Place a large roll behind your baby's back and toys in front to look at. Keep your baby in this position for five to thirty minutes several times a day, when they are calm and awake. Supervise your baby so that they don't fall asleep (this side-lying position is not recommended for sleep). When you pick up your baby, the skin might be a little red or pink from the pressure on the floor (this is like the mark left by a crossed leg). This redness is a good sign, as it means that the pressure from the weight of your baby's head against the floor was effective and will help with reshaping. The redness will be temporary.
- If your baby's flat spots do not resolve, talk to your baby's doctor.

Torticollis

A preference to look to one side and a flat spot on your baby's head may further develop into tight neck muscles on the preferred side. This is referred to as torticollis. Tight neck muscles will limit your baby's neck movement and affect development. Babies with torticollis can look to one side easily but cannot look to the other side very well.

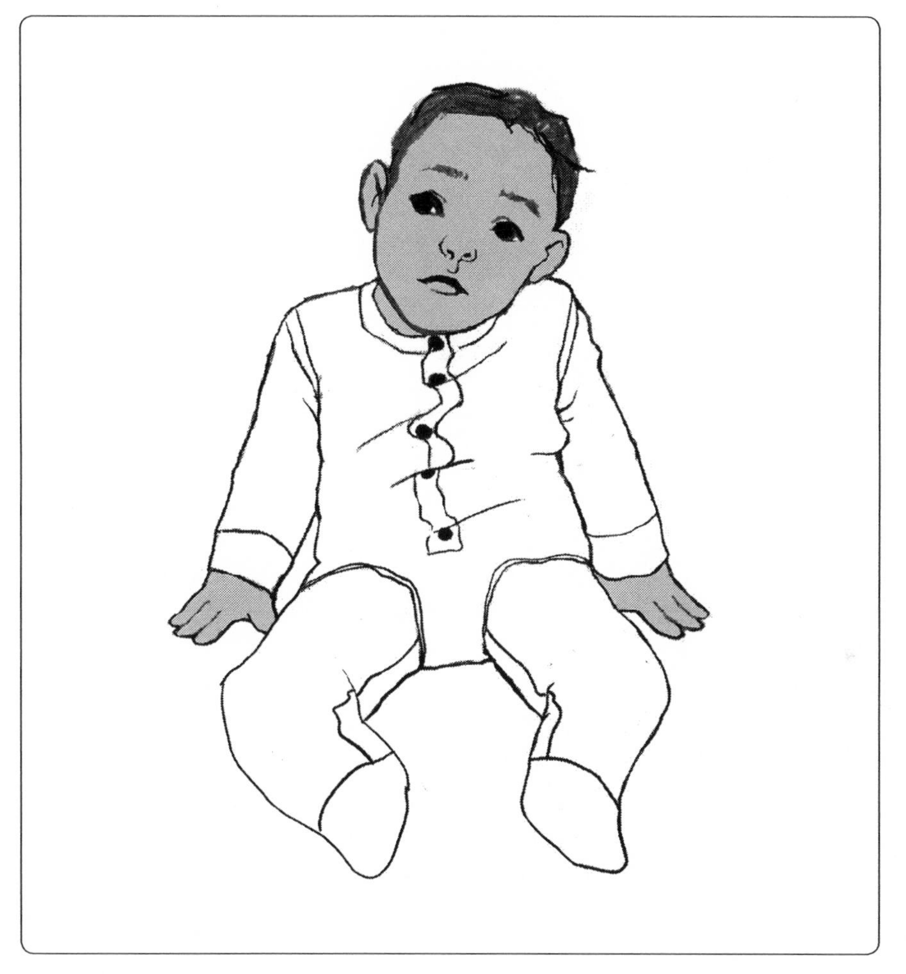

Baby with torticollis.

Torticollis might be more noticeable once your baby is two to four months corrected age. When you hold your baby in seated position, look at how your baby holds their head. If your baby's head tips to one side on a regular basis as shown in the illustration above, this might be torticollis. Another sign of torticollis is resistance (for example, fussing and irritability) when turning their head to one side, especially when turning away from the flattened side of their head.

If you suspect your baby has torticollis, you should see your baby's doctor. The doctor may give you neck stretches to do to lengthen those tight muscles. They may also make a referral to a physiotherapist.

Massage for babies

Baby massage is fairly simple and doesn't require special training. It is a lovely way to connect with your baby. We share some introductory tips below to get you started. For further information, look for baby massage classes in your community or videos online (see our website at www.preemiecare.ca for suggestions).

Massage helps to calm babies by releasing oxytocin, or the "happy" hormone, and promotes sleep, relaxation, brain development, and parent-infant attachment. You will likely also feel relaxed while you massage your baby.

Massage can be done anytime in part or in full. It is best not to do a full body massage right after a feed. In between feeds or after a bath might be enjoyable. You can build a little routine, such as at bed time. Unlike adult massage, the purpose of baby massage is not to knead out muscle knots and muscle strain, but to relax and bond with your baby. If you see that your baby is uncomfortable, restless, or making an unhappy face, slow down or stop. Baby massage should be enjoyable for your baby.

You don't have to use massage oil, as the important thing about massage is the gentle stroking and the special time together. Without oil, you should move your hands and fingers very slowly. Massage oil allows your hands to guide over your baby's skin and prevent friction. If you want to use massage oil, use one that is safe for your baby's skin and for hands in their mouth (in other words, edible and non-toxic). Do not use oils that are made from mineral oil or paraffin.

Mineral oil is a product of petroleum and has many chemicals. Choose oils that are labeled:

- non-scented;
- organic or natural;
- pesticide-free, chemical-free;
- cold-pressed (which means chemicals were not used to make this oil);
- made from fruit or vegetables.

Examples include sesame oil, grapeseed oil, coconut oil, or almond oil. Oils with vitamin E added are good for baby's skin. Olive oil is too thick and can cause baby's skin to dry out. Test the oil first by applying a small amount to one area of your baby's skin and watching for any redness or dryness over two days. If you note a skin reaction, do not use that oil on your baby's skin.

For babies on oxygen, never use oil for massage, as it is a fire hazard. You could use a water-based lotion, but you will find that it absorbs quickly.

ACTION PLAN: Baby Massage

Baby massage is recommended at every developmental stage in the first year (see chapter 6). Here are tips for how to do it:

- Remove your jewelry.
- Breathe deeply and relax before you start.
- Massage in a warm room. To prevent heat loss, cover the other parts of your baby's body with a light blanket.
- If you are comfortable sitting on the floor, lay your baby between your legs facing you. Lean forward from your hips and keep your back straight during the massage. Do not round your back as this can cause muscle strain. If you are prone to back problems, place baby on a table for the massage.
- Lay your baby down on their back, on a towel if you are using oil, and warm up the oil in your hands before touching baby.
- Look at your baby in their eyes. Talk or sing to them. Smile! Skin contact and massage is an expression of love.
- When you start to massage, be very gentle. Massage can be stimulating if done too quickly or too firmly.
- Move your hands slowly and rhythmically, with long gentle strokes. Also try a light, feathery touch on your baby's skin.
- Start on one of your baby's legs. For each leg, start near the hip and wrap your hands around the leg. Slide your hands down to the foot while maintaining a gentle squeeze.
- Hold the foot and massage circles on the top and bottom of the foot.

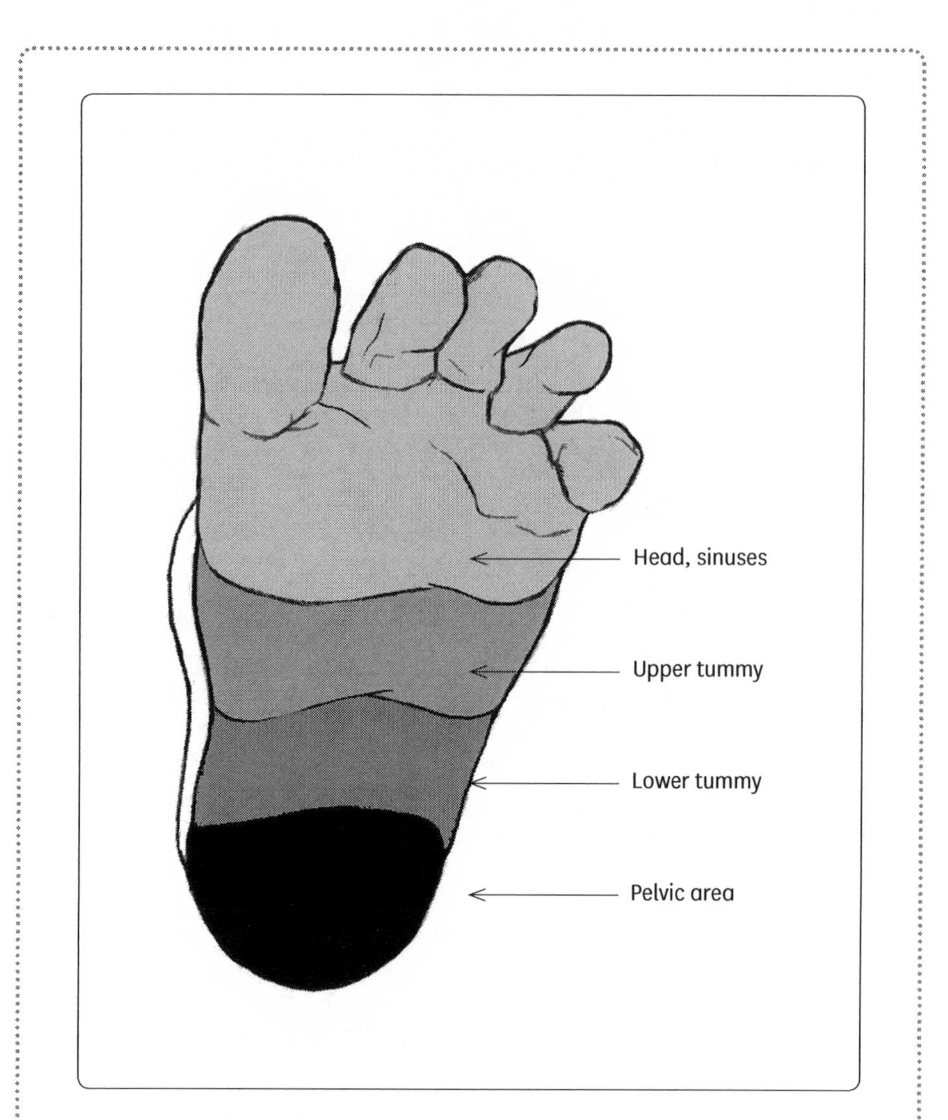

This simplified illustration shows a baby's foot massage zones.

- Slide your fingers down over each toe and give each toe a little squeeze and a little pull.
- Apply gentle pressure on the bottom of the foot to stimulate the thousands of nerve endings there. Reflexology theory claims that foot massage will help comfort other parts of your baby's body and promote overall health (see illustration above).
- Repeat on the other leg.

- Move next to the middle of the body and spread your hands over your baby's chest. Apply gentle pressure as you move upward and over the shoulders and down the arms or to the sides.
- Place your hand over the stomach and gently press while you make clockwise circles with your hand. Your baby might tighten their tummy muscles underneath your hand. This helps digestion. If your baby is gassy, bend your baby's knees up to their stomach and gently hold for thirty seconds or try bicycling the legs, one at a time.
- Stroke the tummy with your fingers, spelling your baby's name or the word "love."
- For each arm, start near the shoulder and wrap your hands around the arm. Slide your hands down while maintaining a gentle squeeze.
- Massage little circles over the top and bottom of each hand. Slide your fingers down each finger, giving each finger a squeeze and a gentle pull.
- Massage your baby's face by placing your hands over the forehead and stroke outward. Run your thumbs down the sides of their nose and out to their ears, around the ears and along their jawbone, ending at the chin.
- And finally, turn your baby over and, with their head turned to one side, massage the back. Massage in circles over the shoulders and down the back. Little circles over your baby's spine will feel nice. Try feathery strokes, too.

Your baby will show you what they like by calming down and what they don't like by fussing or crying. Babies tend to change their minds a lot so keep trying! Soon your baby will learn the routine and will really enjoy this special time you spend together. And, hopefully, have a nice long sleep afterward!

Giving medications

You are responsible for making sure your baby receives the correct medications in the right amount at the scheduled time(s). Some babies require multiple medications. You will be tired and may forget. Parents often ask how to keep track of these medications.

In the first few days, I struggled to keep all my baby's medications sorted out and get the timing right. My husband developed a medication record, like a chart, which helped keep us on track. We kept all the medications in the same place, so they were easy to find.

I drew up all her meds for the day and attached the syringes to the medication bottle with an elastic band. When I looked in the fridge, I saw the syringes and was reminded to give them.

There are tried-and-true strategies that will help ensure oral medications are given safely and as prescribed.

ACTION PLAN: Medications

Try these strategies for oral medications:

- Know the name, purpose, when to give, how much to give, and possible side effects of the medication.
- Know how best to store the medication (some require refrigeration).
- Keep all medications out of the reach of other children.
- Draw up all the medications each morning so you are prepared for the day. Label the medications with tape.
- Post a checklist of when medications are due, perhaps on a small whiteboard.
- Set an alarm on your phone to go off at medication times.
- Do not mix a medication in a full bottle. Your baby may not finish the bottle and you won't know how much medication they actually had.
- If you can give the medication with feeds, put the medication in a bottle with 10 to 20 ml (2 to 4 tsp) of breast milk or formula. Once your baby has taken the medication, continue with the feed.

- For medications that must be given on an empty stomach, ask your baby's doctor or a pharmacist if the medication can be given in 10 to 20 ml (2 to 4 tsp) of breast milk or formula.
- If your baby receives vitamin D drops, give the drop directly into your baby's mouth or onto a soother. Do not mix vitamin D drops into a bottle as the oil-based drop will stick to your baby's bottle.
- Hold your baby securely and comfortably, as this will help both of you stay relaxed and calm.
- Do not give your preemie nonprescription medicines, especially cold or cough medications or syrups, without checking with your doctor.
- Do not give fever medications to a baby younger than three months corrected age without first asking a health care professional to determine the safe dose.
- Never give your baby aspirin (also called acetylsalicylic acid) without a doctor's advice.
- Babies over two to three months corrected age may be able to swallow medications placed in their mouth. Put the tip of the syringe in the corner of your baby's mouth by their cheek and encourage them to suck the medication as you squirt. Do not squirt it into the back of the mouth or throat, as this may make your baby gag or choke.
- Use a bottle nipple or breast shield and squirt the medication into the nipple while your baby sucks and swallows it.
- Ask your doctor what to do if your baby throws up right after given a medication. Most medications should not be repeated.
- If you miss a medication, give it as soon as you remember. Gradually adjust the time of the next doses until you are back on schedule. If you completely forget a dose, do not give two doses at once. Give the next scheduled dose and continue on the schedule.
- If you have trouble giving your baby oral medication, ask your health care provider (doctor, nurse, pharmacist) for advice.

Try these strategies for eye and nose drops:

- Use two people for administering eye or nose drops, if possible. Have one person hold the baby securely while the other gives the drops.
- If you are alone, swaddle your baby with a blanket around their chest.
- For eye drops, lay your baby flat on your lap, holding the head steady and pulling down the lower eyelid. Place one drop in the pocket of the lower lid. Hold the eyelid for the count of five and then release. If you release too soon, your baby will blink out the eye drop.
- Repeat if you need to give more than one drop.
- For nose drops, lay your baby flat on your lap and tilt the head back slightly. Give the required number of drops into each nostril.

Sterilizing bottles, nipples, and water

For full-term newborns, the common recommendation is to sterilize bottles, nipples, and water used to make formula until four months of age. Applying this recommendation to premature newborns, we recommend that you sterilize bottles, nipples, and water for formula until four months corrected age. Beyond this age, a baby's immune system can handle the normal germs in your home and, in fact, it's then healthy for a building immune system to be exposed to the "normal" world. Discontinue sterilizing after four months corrected age unless otherwise directed by your baby's doctor.

Drooling near four months corrected age

Around four months corrected age you will notice that your baby is drooling more. Many parents think this is a sign of teething. However, teething normally occurs closer to six months corrected age.

If your baby's gums are firm and not swollen, and you cannot see or feel teeth, the drooling is likely related to a maturing digestive system. Around four months corrected age, your baby's mouth begins to make saliva. Up until now, your baby did not need to make saliva because breast milk and formula are easy to digest in the stomach. In a couple of months your baby will be swallowing purees made from grains, vegetables, fruits, and meats. To properly digest these foods, our bodies make saliva, which begins to break down food as we chew and swallow.

This saliva collects in your baby's mouth, but your baby does not yet know how to move it from the front to the back of the mouth for swallowing. That's why your baby is drooling. Saliva is full of digestive enzymes, so you might notice your baby's chin and become red or irritated. While we can't stop the drooling, we can prevent skin irritation.

ACTION PLAN: Drooling

Try these strategies for drooling:

- Frequently wipe drool off your baby's face, using a warm facecloth rather than baby wipes, paper towels, or irritating soap. Wipe their neck and neck folds. Pat skin gently with a soft towel.
- Use baby bibs when your baby is supervised. Remove bib when baby is sleeping to avoid strangulation.
- Give your baby a bottle, finger, soother, or breast to suck, which will clear the mouth of saliva.
- If your baby's skin is red or irritated by drool, clean more frequently. Apply a thin layer of organic, chemical-free barrier cream that is safe for babies, as your baby will be touching their chin and then putting their hands in their mouth.

Teething and premature babies

Teething usually occurs close to six months corrected age but could occur between four months and one year corrected age. Usually the bottom two teeth come first. For some babies, many teeth grow in at once. Others sprout one a time.

There are several symptoms of teething:

- swollen, soft gums;
- teeth you can feel or see protruding through gums;
- excessive drooling;
- biting, chewing, or gnawing on toys;
- flushed cheeks (for some babies);
- irritability, increased crying, need of more comfort, not eating as well as usual, waking more during the night.

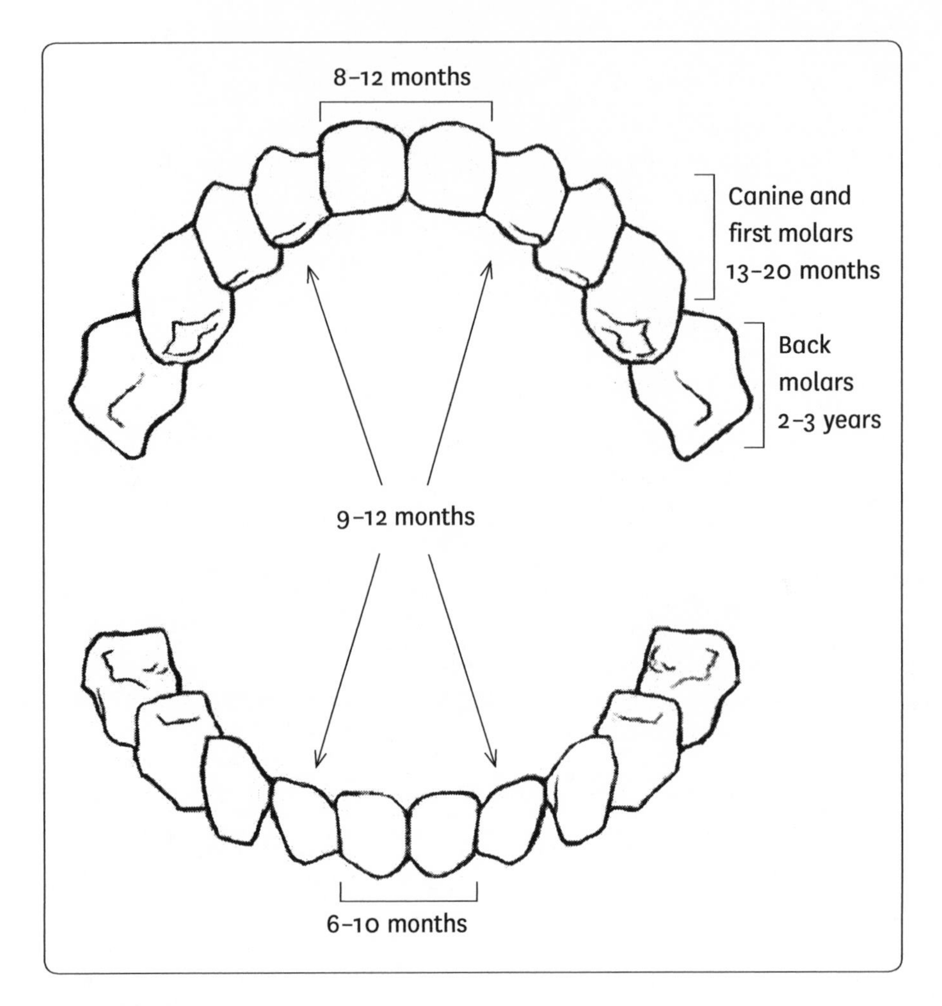

Chart of typical teeth eruption.

Parents of teething babies should provide comfort care. If you are concerned about your baby's teeth, contact your baby's doctor. Book an appointment with your dentist about six months after the first tooth erupts or around one year corrected age.

ACTION PLAN: Teething

Try these strategies for teething:

- Provide safe toys to chew on. Your baby might like toys that are hard or bumpy or to chew on a baby toothbrush (no toothpaste). Leave these in the fridge so they are nice and cool to bite on.
- Make sure the liquid inside baby's teething ring is water and therefore the ring would be safe if it were to rupture. (Read the label.)
- Do not freeze teething rings. The frozen ring could cause skin or mouth damage.
- With your finger or a cool, wet cloth, gently rub your baby's gums for several minutes.
- Moisten a cloth with water and freeze. Let your baby bite on the cold cloth.
- Give your baby smaller and more frequent feeds.
- Give your baby extra attention and hold them more often. Be patient! This will pass soon.
- If your baby's skin is irritated by drool, follow the strategies in the action plan for drooling above.
- Do not use teething gels, which contain an anesthetic. These could put your baby at risk for choking, if the anesthetic reaches the back of the throat. Teething gels may also contain chemicals that are not good for babies. Ask your doctor's advice about teething gels.
- Avoid teething necklaces. There is no evidence that they work and they are a choking risk.
- If your baby is over six months corrected age and has been already eaten purees, try feeding them a cool puree.
- If your baby is in pain, you can give acetaminophen/paracetamol.

Special Care for Babies Who Become Sick

In this section we will review common signs of illness and parent strategies for when baby seems sick. We hope you never need this information, but it's best to know what to look for and to be prepared.

Signs of illness

Watch for several signs of illness:

- Breathing sixty or more times a minute that does not slow down when your baby is calm.
- Increased breathing effort, anxious expression, increased indrawing.
- Noisy breathing, such as wheezing or high-pitched crowing sounds.
- Not breathing.
- Temperature under 36°C (96.8°F) and it does not increase after skin-to-skin cuddle or adding extra layer of clothing.
- Temperature over 38°C (100.4°F) and it does not decrease after removing extra layers.
- Decreased urine output; dry diapers; increased thirst; no tears; dry skin, mouth, and tongue.
- Diarrhea.
- Vomiting the full feed two or more times in a row.
- Not feeding as well without apparent causes, such as overstimulation, busy appointment day, vaccinations, or eye examination in last twenty-four hours.
- Lethargy or not waking up.
- Irritability that will not decrease when comforted.
- Baby seems to be in pain.
- Blood in bowel movement.
- Hard, distended abdomen.
- Cyanosis (blue color), pale color.

How you should respond to these signs depends on the symptom severity and how unwell your baby looks. If your baby has a mild symptom, such as not eating as well as usual, you might choose to observe for a couple of hours. If your baby had a fever but their temperature came down when you removed a blanket, you might choose to wait to see what happens. If your baby vomited twice and looks pale but is otherwise acting normally, you might choose to drive your baby to the doctor's office in the next one to two hours. If your baby has blood in the bowel movement or a hard abdomen, your baby needs medical attention urgently. If your baby is not breathing, start rescue breathing and call for an ambulance. When in doubt about your baby's symptoms of illness, you should seek an assessment by a doctor. Trust your parental instinct.

Strategies for increased breathing effort

Premature babies are at higher risk of respiratory illness and rehospitalization in the first year of life. Watch your baby closely for respiratory distress.

If you see increased breathing effort, rule out other causes and try our suggestions to ease the breathing effort:

- Look for other signs of illness, for example, check your baby's temperature and color, and count your baby's breathing rate for one minute.
- Assess whether your baby in pain or discomfort.
- Offer a feed to assess whether your baby is upset due to hunger.
- Note whether your baby just finished crying or straining, for example, from a big bowel movement. If so, recheck breathing once they calm down.
- Check if your baby's nostrils are congested. If so, attempt to clear.
- Hold baby upright against you, chest to chest, and recheck breathing effort.
- Offer a soother to calm.

If your baby has other signs of illness or if breathing effort does not ease with calming, seek medical advice from a doctor.

Strategies for low temperature

A low temperature (under 36˚C; 98.6˚F) could be the result if your baby is not dressed warmly enough, has minimal skin fat, or is unable to maintain a normal temperature due to sickness.

Try these strategies to bring your baby's temperature back to normal:

- Do skin-to-skin contact, with baby lying on your chest, wearing only a diaper, with a cozy blanket covering their back. This is the most effective way to rewarm your baby. Recheck baby's temperature in twenty to thirty minutes.

- Dress baby in more layers. Bundle in a blanket. Recheck baby's temperature in twenty to thirty minutes.

- Look for other signs of illness, for example, breathing rate and effort and skin color.

- Seek medical advice from a doctor if temperature does not return to normal range or if other signs of illness are present. In particular, babies under three months corrected age should usually be seen by a doctor if low temperature or signs of illness continue. These babies are at greater risk of infection and dehydration.

Strategies for high temperature

A high temperature (over 38°C; 100.4°F) could occur if your baby is overdressed, has had a vaccination or is sick.

Try these strategies to bring your baby's temperature back to normal:

- Remove layers of clothing and recheck temperature in twenty to thirty minutes.
- Never put cold cloths on your baby.
- Look for other signs of illness, such as diarrhea or low urine output.
- See a doctor right away if your baby has a temperature over 38°C and is under three months corrected age. Do not give fever medication unless advised by a doctor.
- If your baby is over three months corrected age, give acetaminophen/paracetamol as directed for your baby's corrected age and weight. Recheck temperature thirty minutes after giving acetaminophen/paracetamol.
- If your baby feels warm but has a temperature under 38°C (100.4°F), give comfort care, and continue to monitor for fever. Do not give fever medication if your baby's temperature is under 38°C. Your baby's body raises the body temperature in an effort to fight off infection. By suppressing the warmer temperature, you could be allowing the virus to get stronger.
- If temperature does not return to normal range or if other signs of illness are present, seek medical advice from a doctor. Younger babies under three months corrected age, who are at a greater risk of infection and dehydration, should be seen by a doctor if high temperature or signs of illness continue.

Don't give your young baby repeated doses of fever medication, as these can mask the signs of infection and make your baby sleepy and not interested in feeding. Meanwhile the infection can get worse. Take your baby to a doctor if fever persists.

Strategies for dehydration

Dehydration is the loss of body fluids without adequate replacement. Dehydration can occur very quickly in young babies. If not resolved, dehydration can lead to organ failure and death. Dehydration in babies is most often caused by either diarrhea, vomiting, and/or poor intake. You will find more strategies to address low intake strategies in chapter 4, and diarrhea and vomiting in chapter 5.

Signs of dehydration include:

- decreased wet diapers (less than four wet diapers in twenty-four hours or no wet diaper in six hours);
- absence of tears;
- dry, cool skin;
- dry, sticky mouth and tongue;
- sunken eyes;
- pale or gray skin color;
- behavior change (irritable, drowsy, sleepy);
- sunken soft spot (fontanel) on head;

Babies under three months corrected age are at particular risk of dehydration. If your baby shows any of the above signs of dehydration, take your baby to a doctor or emergency department.

Babies over three months corrected age are at less risk of dehydration and have stronger immune systems to fight the viruses that cause vomiting and diarrhea. Many of these viruses last twenty-four hours. The goal of care is to keep your baby well hydrated in the meantime.

The following are a few things you can do:

- Continue to feed your baby as usual. If you are giving breast milk and formula, try giving only breast milk until the symptoms abate. Breast milk is very healing to a baby's gut.
- Look for other signs of illness, such as fever, refusal to take liquids, no urine output for six hours, lethargy.
- Ask your baby's doctor about small, frequent feeds of electrolyte solutions. These solutions are designed for babies and available in drugstores/pharmacies.
- If other symptoms of illness are present or if the diarrhea and/or vomiting do not subside, seek medical advice from a doctor.

All parents worry when their baby gets sick. The first time can be hard on parents. Watch your baby for all signs of illness and monitor if your baby is getting better or worse. If you continue to see no improvement, seek medical advice from a doctor. In cases of medical emergency, always head for your closest emergency department or phone for an ambulance, such as 911.

Special Care for Babies on Oxygen at Home

A term baby is born with up to 150 million air sacs in the lungs, called "alveoli." These air sacs are where the lungs exchange carbon dioxide and oxygen. A very premature baby will have fewer alveoli at birth and these sacs are stiffer, prone to collapse, and less effective in oxygen–carbon dioxide gas exchange. The lungs of babies are able to produce new alveoli to promote healing over time.

Bronchopulmonary dysplasia (BPD), or chronic lung disease, commonly occurs in preterm or low birth weight babies who require mechanical ventilation and oxygen therapy. BPD is characterized by structural changes in the lungs that result from prematurity and the necessary treatments to keep premature babies alive. The more premature the baby, the greater the risk for BPD.

If your baby has been diagnosed with BPD, your baby might:

- have a faster breathing rate;
- show some indrawing with breathing;
- have less energy reserve;
- be easily overstimulated;
- need oxygen at home;
- need more calories for healing and lung growth;
- need extra feeding strategies to avoid compromised breathing;
- be more susceptible to viruses (colds) and nasal congestion;
- be more likely to be hospitalized with respiratory infection.

Most babies with BPD recover completely, but some have long-term respiratory health issues. Lung healing and growth are optimized by preventing illness and paying attention to good nutrition and growth.

Giving oxygen to a baby at home

Supplemental oxygen is usually delivered through nasal prongs or "cannula"—a small tube that fits under your baby's nose and around the head. Three types of oxygen delivery systems may be used in the home:

1. **Compressed gas.** Oxygen gas is pressurized into cylinders or tanks. The length of time between cylinder changes depends on how much oxygen your baby uses and on the size of the tank. You should have several small tanks for traveling with your baby.

2. **Oxygen concentrator (like a small, noisy fridge).** An oxygen concentrator is a device that separates oxygen from the air and gives it to your baby. The concentrator provides a continuous supply of oxygen and there is no need for replacing cylinders. Because a concentrator runs on electricity, a portable backup oxygen tank is needed for when your baby is away from home or in the event of a power outage. One drawback of an oxygen concentrator is that it may be noisy and it releases heat, which can make a room too warm.

3. **Liquid oxygen.** This is oxygen that has been cooled to a liquid state and that changes to a gas as your baby breathes it. Sometimes, portable tanks may be filled from a larger tank. One drawback of liquid oxygen is that it evaporates when not in use. Ask your oxygen company how long the portable and main tank should last. Liquid oxygen is also expensive and may not be covered by health insurance.

Precautions for oxygen at home

Regardless of the type of oxygen system in your home, certain safety measures must be followed. Because oxygen is a highly flammable substance there are certain precautions you need to take.

ACTION PLAN: Home Oxygen Use

Try these strategies for safe home oxygen use:

- Don't smoke in the home or around the oxygen.
- When your baby is receiving oxygen, do not use open flames, such as from heaters, fireplaces, or gas appliances with pilot lights.
- Do not use an open flame, such as a candle, in a room with oxygen.
- Do not use rubbing alcohol, oil, petroleum jelly, electric razors, or aerosol spray cans near a baby on oxygen.
- Keep the door to your baby's room open, so the room is well ventilated.
- Ensure the smoke detectors in your home work well.
- Periodically review your home fire escape plan with your family.

Caring for a baby on home oxygen

Normally, when babies are ready to go home, they are very stable with the prescribed oxygen flow rate and don't need an oxygen saturation monitor or "pulse oximeter" (a machine that measures the percentage of oxygen attached to your baby's red blood cells). Pulse oximeters are known for frequent false alarms, especially when a baby is active, which limits their usefulness in the home setting. Non-medical-grade baby monitors designed as socks or mattress pads are unreliable, expensive, and, in our experience, quickly abandoned by parents after trying them out. Most oxygen-dependent babies will have their oxygenation measured periodically by a respiratory care practitioner in the home or at a clinic.

The best way to monitor your baby is by observation. In time, you will become a good judge of your baby's breathing and be able to detect any changes. Get to know your baby's baseline respiratory status.

Know your baby's normal:

- respiratory rate (number of breaths per minute);
- color;
- breathing sounds;
- breathing effort.

If you are concerned about your baby's breathing, turn up the oxygen. If you see an improvement, contact your baby's doctor or respiratory specialist for further advice.

! **Take your baby to the nearest emergency department if baby exhibits:**

- fast breathing that does not settle when baby is calm;
- increased breathing effort;
- increased indrawing of the chest or neck, and flaring of the nostrils;
- grunting, wheezing, or high-pitched crowing sounds;
- paler than usual color that does not improve with increase in oxygen flow;
- restlessness or agitation;
- more sleepy than usual and lack of responsiveness to arousal;
- a lot of irritability or fussiness and cannot be comforted;
- inability to feed or drink;
- dehydration. (This means your child's body does not have enough fluid to work properly and can happen when your baby is not drinking enough. Signs of dehydration include dry or sunken eyes and decreased urination.)

Call 911 if your baby is blue, not breathing, or having trouble breathing. If your baby is not breathing, give mouth-to-mouth rescue breathing until the ambulance arrives. If your baby does not have a pulse, start infant CPR.

ACTION PLAN: Baby on Oxygen

Try these strategies for care of your baby on oxygen:

- Place socks on your baby's hands for sleep times to prevent your baby from removing the prongs. Socks will stay on longer than hand mitts.
- Place a strip of tape over the nasal prongs and onto your baby's nose to secure the tubing when you are not supervising them.

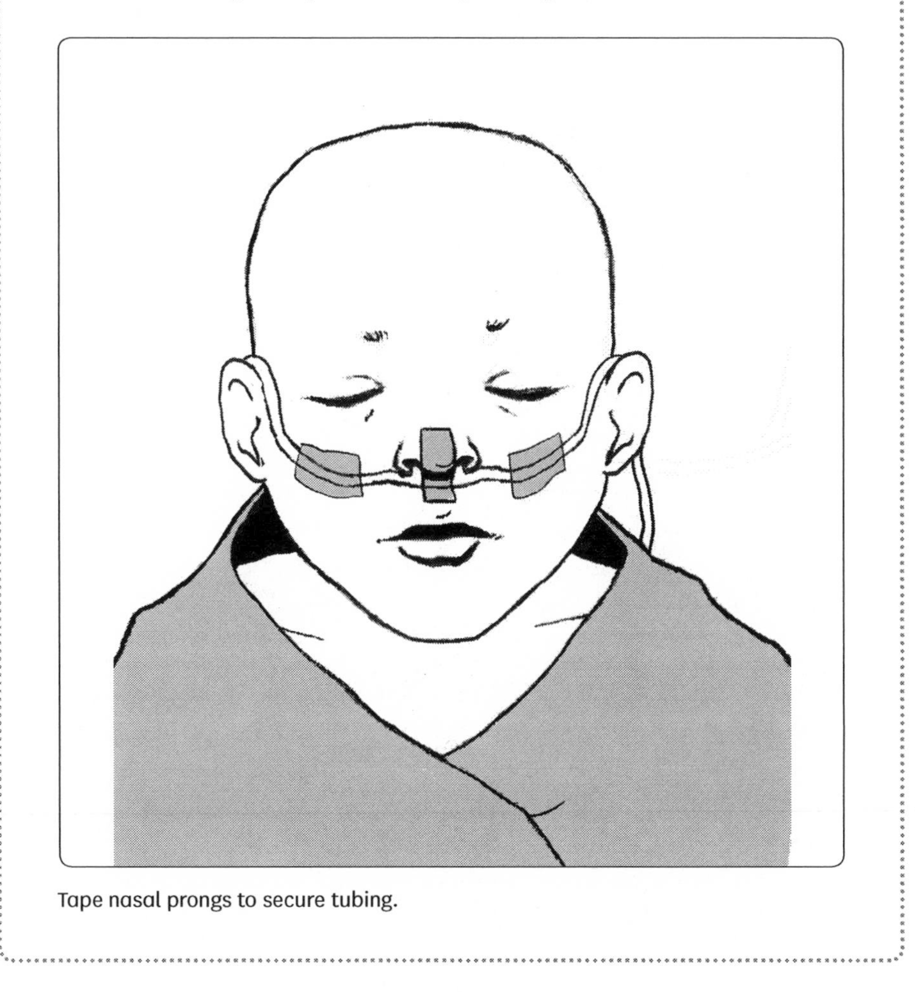

Tape nasal prongs to secure tubing.

- Choose a stroller with the biggest possible basket to hold the oxygen tank.
- Ask for long extension tubing (fifty feet) to be able to move around the house.
- If you have an oxygen concentrator, place in a room adjacent to the one where baby sleeps to avoid heating up that room.
- For two-story homes, ask for two tanks—one for upstairs, one for downstairs.
- Change nasal prongs weekly, or more frequently if baby is congested or has milk come up the nose.
- Change the extension tubing as directed.
- Keep extra parts handy (nasal prongs, connectors, tubing) at home and in the car and bring spares with you when you travel.
- If you have other small children in your home, turn the oxygen system to face the wall so that inquisitive fingers cannot adjust the oxygen flow. Tape a paper cup over the flow dial. Place the oxygen system where children cannot access the flow meter (in a closet or off-limits room).
- We recommend humidification of your baby's oxygen; discuss with your oxygen company.
- Use temporary wall hooks to suspend oxygen tubing to prevent tripping hazard. Be careful with tubing on stairs.
- Contact your local neonatal or pediatric unit for a nurse or aide, a nursing school for a student, or a parent support group for a babysitter to care for a healthier baby in a home setting, as an alternative to daycare. Daycares usually don't accept babies on oxygen and it is better to avoid the exposure to germs at these centers.
- You may qualify for caregiver relief support at home. Check with your baby's doctor, community nurse, respiratory specialists, or social workers to see if this is available.
- Keep pets away from tubing by suspending it off the floor.

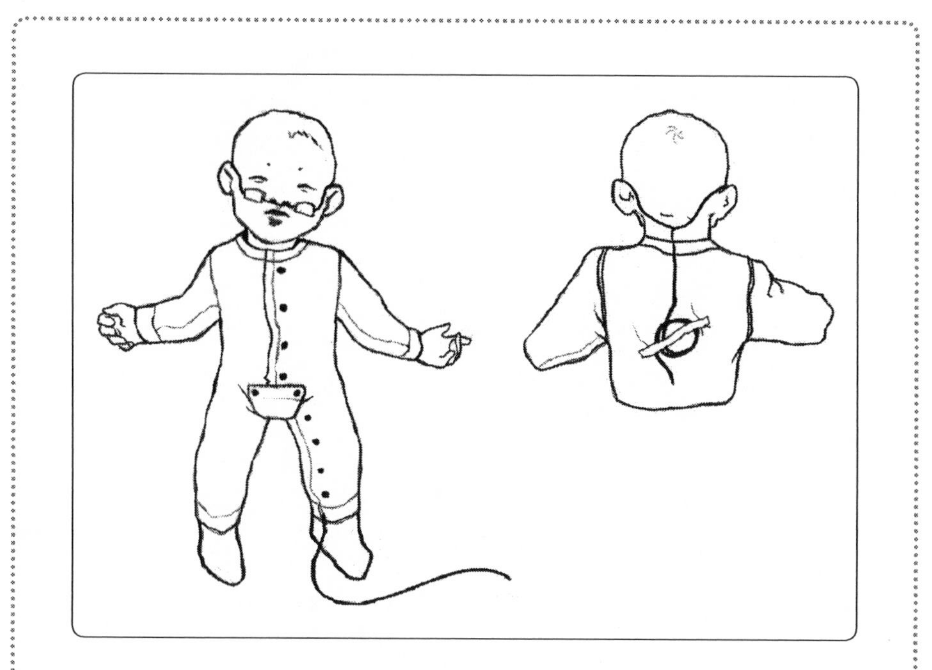

Two methods of securing oxygen tubes.

- Secure the oxygen tubing to ensure the tubing does not wrap around your baby's body or neck during sleep. Refer to the illustrations above to see two methods of securing the oxygen tubing. These techniques are particularly useful once your baby is able to roll over. Follow the illustration on the left and dress your baby in a one-piece, long-legged outfit. Run the tube under the clothing and let it out at the last snap or button on the leg at the ankle. The second method is shown in the illustration on the right. Curl the tubing in a circle and tape it to the back of your baby's clothing. Remember to unfasten the tubing when you remove your baby's outfit.

Balancing life with a baby on oxygen

If your baby needs oxygen, you can still go out, taking the portable oxygen cylinders with you in a backpack or shoulder bag. You can go the park, to appointments, and to visit family and friends. This might sound scary, and you might want help going out for the first few times, but parents adjust to having their baby on oxygen very quickly.

The oxygen doesn't need to be a barrier. All it takes is a little preparation.

ACTION PLAN: Trips with Oxygen

Try these strategies for safer, easier trips out with oxygen:

- Always make sure that the portable tank is turned on before connecting your baby.
- Ensure the tank is full enough for your entire outing.
- Double and triple check that the tubing remains connected and that the oxygen is set to the correct amount (it can move around in transport).
- Carry extra tape, scissors, and tubing.
- Secure the oxygen tank so that it will not move in your vehicle.
- Bring a spare portable oxygen tank in case of emergencies.
- Once you are back home, turn on the home oxygen system before connecting your baby.

While going out with your baby on oxygen is possible, parents must always consider the risk of infection. Review the section "Protection from sickness" at the beginning of this chapter. Protecting babies with fragile lungs is crucial to avoiding illness and rehospitalization.

Follow-up appointments

Most babies on oxygen receive follow-up from an outpatient clinic that specializes in home oxygen therapy. These clinics often have a full multidisciplinary team, including a physiotherapist, dietitian, doctor, nurse, and oral feeding specialist (occupational or speech-language therapist). Home nursing visits may be recommended based on your baby's health needs, your health care coverage, and availability in your community.

Oxygen weaning

The decision to begin weaning a baby from oxygen depends on many factors. Sometimes the weaning process is started when the baby's respiratory effort decreases and oxygen saturation stabilizes. This is typically when the lungs have begun to heal. Other babies stay on oxygen to support optimal weight gain and attainment of developmental milestones.

Do not lower the oxygen flow rate unless the doctor tells you to. Sometimes parents might be tempted to turn off or lower the oxygen because their baby looks fine.

> *My baby was pulling the tubing from his nose, so I told my doctor that my baby didn't like the oxygen and was ready to come off. My doctor told me that taking the oxygen off too soon could hurt my baby's lungs and brain and that the true measure of being ready to come off oxygen was the oxygen saturation test.*

Turning down or discontinuing the oxygen may cause a slowing of your baby's growth or injury to your baby's lungs, heart, or brain. Even if your baby doesn't turn blue on lower oxygen, do not lower the oxygen unless advised by a doctor. Our eyes are not as reliable as medical equipment as a test for oxygen levels. Studies report fewer respiratory infections in babies on oxygen than in those whose oxygen saturation levels are borderline.

In determining when to wean the oxygen, your doctor will consider many factors unique to your baby. Past history, test results, health, and growth will be considered. Doctors may be more cautious with weaning during the colder winter months when lots of viruses are present. Weaning is usually gradual and is accompanied by physical examinations, chest X-rays, and periodic oxygenation measurements. Your baby's doctor or clinical team will explain the weaning process for your baby. One way to wean is to take babies off oxygen for several hours a day. Another is to leave the oxygen off when baby's awake and put it back on for sleep. If babies fail to progress in the weaning schedule, they are evaluated to determine the cause. To support weaning, the best thing to keep your baby healthy and growing well. And be patient. Lung healing takes time.

Final Thoughts

Even with the high risk of rehospitalization in the first year, most premature babies sail through this period without readmission to hospital. Nevertheless, sometimes babies become sick despite the diligent care from their parents and extended family. You can't protect your baby from all viruses. But you can help reduce the risk.

♥ *It all began so subtly. She was more tired and not eating as well as usual. I thought it was because we'd had a busy day. But she didn't perk up the next day, was still not eating well, and then I noticed her diapers were lighter. I checked her temperature a few times and it was always normal. She looked pale and tired. Then the cold symptoms kicked in—stuffy nose, heavy breathing, and coughing. I took her to emergency and they admitted her. A respiratory virus, they said. She had to go back on oxygen, which upset me a lot. I thought that was all behind us. She was in for about six days and off oxygen and eating okay by then. That bad lingering cough would make her throw up after feeds. Our nurse gave us anti-reflux suggestions, like small frequent feeds and holding her upright afterward. It took a couple weeks to settle down.*

After spending 105 days in the NICU, the last place we wanted to go was back into hospital. We don't know how she caught that virus. No one else in our family was sick. And we didn't take her anywhere there were sick people. We did everything we could to protect her. Thankfully, that was the only trip back to hospital she had in more than two years.

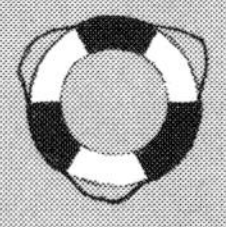

EXPERT TIPS

Here are the key strategies to navigate the journey

- Know the signs and symptoms of illness.
- Avoid sick people.
- Avoid smoke.
- Vaccinate your baby.
- Wash hands frequently to minimize your baby's exposure to germs.
- Create a safe sleeping environment.
- Monitor your baby's head shape.
- Have fun with baby massage.
- Give medications as prescribed.
- Follow the strategies for babies on home oxygen.

4

FUELING UP
Feeding and Growth

ASK ANY parent of a premature baby and they will tell you that the hardest part of care at home is feeding. Some premature babies lack the strength, endurance, or coordination to feed successfully. Ideal goals of breastfeeding may clash with the reality of optimizing growth. How much your baby drinks may conflict with how much the health care team says is needed. Thus many parents of premature babies struggle with the workload of breastfeeding, bottle feeding, and pumping breast milk.

In this chapter, we have tried to address every question and concern parents of premature babies have raised with us about feeding, from strategies for breastfeeding to bottle feeding to tube feeding to spoon feeding, so that you can troubleshoot when your baby is not feeding well. We provide suggestions to help make feedings enjoyable and successful and avoid the pitfalls the following mother experienced:

♥ *I thought we were ready for discharge and, for the most part, we were. We practiced everything from diaper changes to temperature-taking to breastfeeding and bottle feeding. We listened to what the nurses told us and we practiced. But the part that was the hardest—what blew us away—was how hard feeding was.*

After going home, she stopped breastfeeding altogether, as though she forgot how. And then she started falling asleep after taking only half a bottle. I felt like a failure. Why couldn't I do this when it seemed so easy for the NICU nurses? I was so scared she wasn't going to gain weight and would have be readmitted to hospital.

I had to let go of breastfeeding. I didn't know if she was getting anything. I knew that breast milk was the best for her, but at least she was getting breast milk in her bottle. Even then, pumping enough was getting harder. So, I did the only thing I could. I made her take more from the bottle. I felt bad doing it because she was so tired. I sent my mom out to buy other nipples that she might take more from. I think we tried six or seven different ones. None of them worked. She just spilled all over herself and coughed and choked and cried.

Feeding Essentials

The challenge of feeding premature babies

While full-term newborns seem to figure out how to feed by breast or bottle, babies born prematurely need time to learn to feed, develop feeding skills, and become strong enough to fully feed by themselves. There is no magic switch that turns on at term. Waiting until babies are older is not the solution to becoming a good feeder. The learning process is challenging for premature babies.

Your baby may still be premature at the time of discharge. The work on feeding coordination and efficiency continues long after NICU discharge.

Medical problems cause delays. Some babies may take longer to learn to feed because they had medical problems in the NICU (such as necrotizing enterocolitis) or still have medical conditions (such as chronic lung disease).

Communication about feeding is difficult. Your baby may be having trouble telling you about the feeding process. Over time, premature babies learn to give signs when they are ready to start and stop feeding. Your baby will become better at communicating about hunger, feeling full, tummy upset, and the feeding process. When you listen to these cues, feeding will be pleasurable for your baby and your baby will continue to be interested in feeding. If you don't listen to these cues, then your baby will learn that feeding is unpleasant and scary.

Feeding is hard work. Feeding for a baby is like exercising. Their heart and breathing rate and effort increases. Some premature babies have low amounts of energy in reserve to feed for very long. Some babies fall asleep during feeds or lose the energy for coordination and start to cough or spill.

Suck-swallow-breathe coordination is challenging. Consider the skill it takes to suck, swallow, and breathe. Think about what you do with a water bottle and straw when you are very thirsty. You suck the liquid into your mouth and swallow repeatedly. Are you breathing? No! You stop sucking and swallowing to take a breath. Your baby will learn to suck, swallow, and breathe in a coordinated pattern. While they are learning to feed, most babies forget this coordination and might not suck or swallow frequently enough, or might forget to breathe. Now the feed can become messy, scary, or unsafe.

One criterion for discharge is a baby's ability to feed safely and effectively. But that doesn't mean that learning to feed is done. Many babies forget how to feed well from time to time. They might be tired or feel unwell. Maybe their tongue and other mouth muscle coordination is changing. Learning to feed is a long process. Watch your baby while feeding to ensure your baby is "keeping it all together" and feeding well.

Special feeding strategies for premature babies

Feeding is a big challenge for most babies born prematurely. Special strategies, performed consistently, help your baby's feeding experience be as safe and pleasant as possible.

The pace and length of the feed needs to be just right. Feeds should not be too fast or too rushed. Your baby needs the right flow rate and to be able to balance breathing with sucking and swallowing. A fast feed might cause breath-holding or inadequate breathing, because the milk is coming too fast. Or it might mean that your baby's stomach fills too quickly, leaving your baby uncomfortable and sleepless (and you, too!). On the other hand, a slow feed is also not ideal. Your baby might lose interest, fall asleep, not drink enough, and be at risk of dehydration and poor growth. You want the feed to last about fifteen to thirty minutes and be enjoyable, not stressful. We will suggest many ways to promote an optimal feeding pace and length.

Breastfeeding a premature baby takes time and effort. Before leaving the NICU, you may have begun pumping your breast milk to keep up a good supply. Once your baby is home, you will be able to work on breastfeeding and take advantage of when your baby seems interested. Keep in mind that babies who are learning to breastfeed are great pretenders. They look like they are breastfeeding, but in fact, they are not transferring enough breast milk. We offer tips to help with positioning, milk transfer, and breastfeeding in this chapter.

Bottle feeding a premature baby can be complex. Compared with babies born full term, premature babies take more time to develop bottle-feeding expertise. Suck coordination, suck strength, and energy levels need to increase. Premature babies might be challenged by breathing or stomach issues. As well, which nipple/bottle system you use can make a big difference for premature babies in bottle-feeding and dual breast-and-bottle-feeding success.

♥ *It is definitely hard for her to breathe and eat—the whole coordination part—but with what the nurses taught us, she is figuring it out. Actually, she has become a much better eater at home. I think it's because only her mom and I feed her.*

Special strategies will help your baby trust, enjoy, and learn to feed safely.

♥ *We found our little niche for how, when, and where to feed him. Eventually I loved feeding my boy. Once I figured out how he wanted to be fed, it was pretty easy. Feeding was our bonding time. His mom would go nap or pump. The house was quiet and we stared into one another's eyes while he fed. That's when I fell in love. I treasured those cuddles.*

We offer an extensive range of strategies to promote feeding success in general, and breastfeeding and bottle feeding in particular. These recommendations will ensure your baby learns to feed in an optimally supportive environment. As your baby learns to master feeding skills, you will notice that you will spend less time on feeding strategies and ultimately that it will become a normal, stress-free part of your daily routine.

Where to feed your baby

Your baby may have spent a lot of time in a noisy, bright neonatal intensive care unit. This setting is very distracting and makes it hard for babies and parents to concentrate. Now that your baby is home, you can control the light and sound levels of your home. See how your baby reacts to different environments, such as the dark and quiet of your bedroom compared with the hustle and bustle of your kitchen. Some babies don't seem to be affected by noise and light, and others will find them troubling during feedings. You might notice that your baby does not feed as much, might be distracted or less coordinated, takes longer to feed, startles often, or cries. These might be signs that you need to control the environment for your baby's feedings. A semi-dark, quiet room is a great place for babies learning to feed. Babies can concentrate on the work of feeding and you can pay closer attention to their needs.

You might have used a pillow to feed your baby in the NICU. Pillows are helpful for feedings. Some mothers like using a breastfeeding pillow and some prefer using a flat pillow. Experiment with which pillow supports your baby in the best position for feeding and feels comfortable for you. Even bottle-fed babies will be more relaxed during feeds if lying on a pillow on your lap. We highly recommend you use a pillow for both breast and bottle feedings. You will see your baby nestle comfortably into the pillow as their body is supported from head to toe. You baby will feed better when feeling secure.

Optimal position for feeds

Whether your baby is breastfeeding or bottle feeding, we recommend a side-lying, or cross cradle, position on a pillow with head slightly above hips.

You might think side-lying position is only for breastfeeding, but babies fed in side-lying position for bottle feeding also have higher oxygen levels and more stable breathing rates and heart rates. When your baby is side-lying, they have better control of the volume of milk in their mouth. If their mouth is too full, either because they are taking big swallows or not swallowing frequently enough, the excess milk will dribble out the corner of their mouth. If they were on their back, the mouthful might make them choke. In addition, nipple bottles drip when they are tipped downward, which can cause pooling in the back of your baby's mouth. This might occur when your baby is pausing or taking a breath and might cause choking.

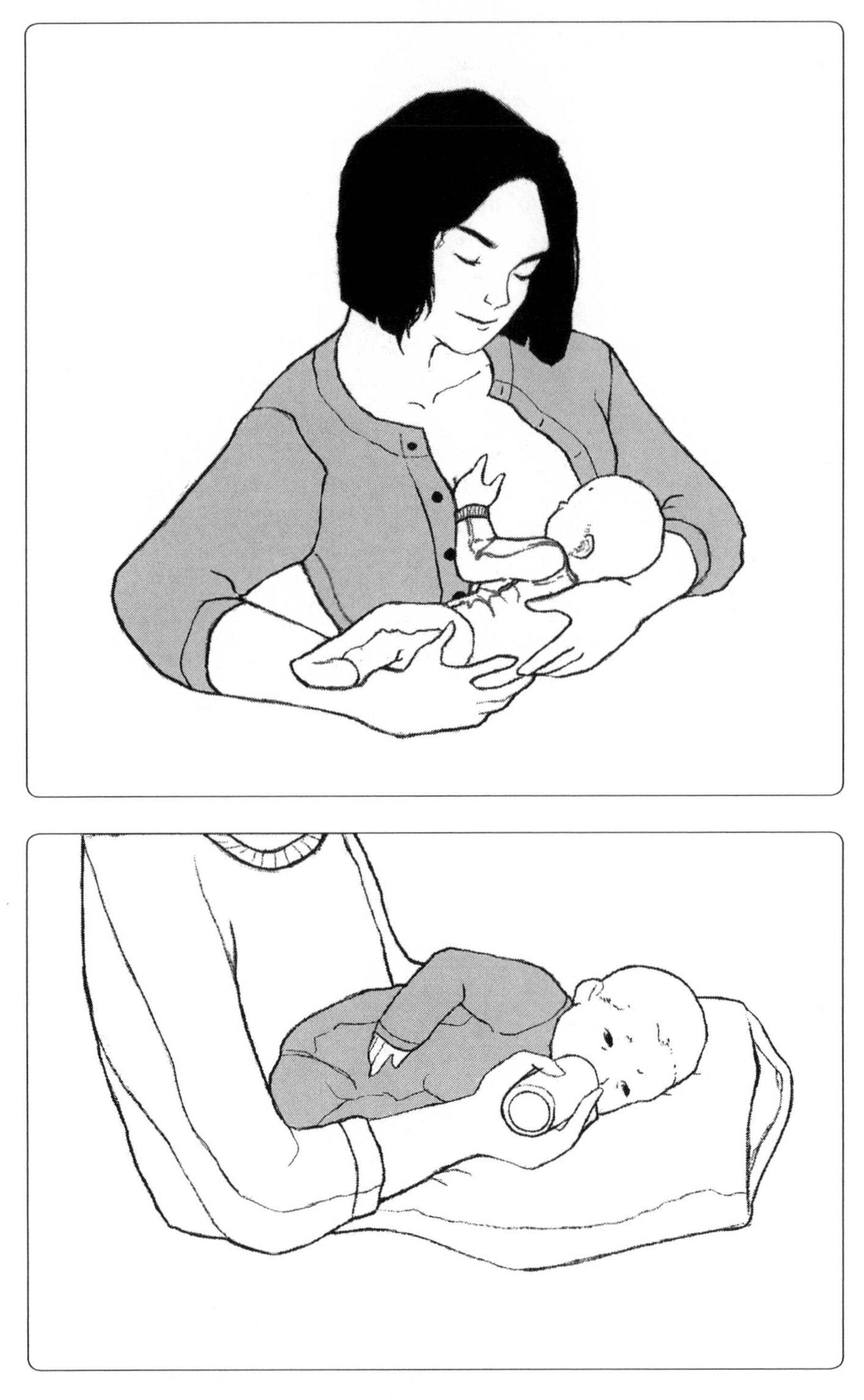

Two side-lying positions for feeds.

Even if you did not try the side-lying position for bottle feeding in hospital, try it with your baby at home. Look closely at the figure above and follow these instructions. Place the pillow across your lap and lay your baby on the side with their bum against your stomach (baby will be at a ninety-degree angle from your body). Raise your feet on a stool so that your baby's head is higher than the body. Lay your baby fully on their side, with that side's ear, shoulder, and hip on the pillow. Don't let your baby slide onto their back into a flat position. A good check is to look for your baby's nose and breastbone to be facing the same direction. Their hips and elbows should be relaxed and slightly bent. Their nose should be slightly raised, similar to a "sniffing position" like the minor lift we reflexively do when we smell something pleasant. Rest your hand and arm on the pillow in front of your baby as you hold the bottle. With your other arm, provide support along your baby's back. This position will allow you to see your baby's face during the feed.

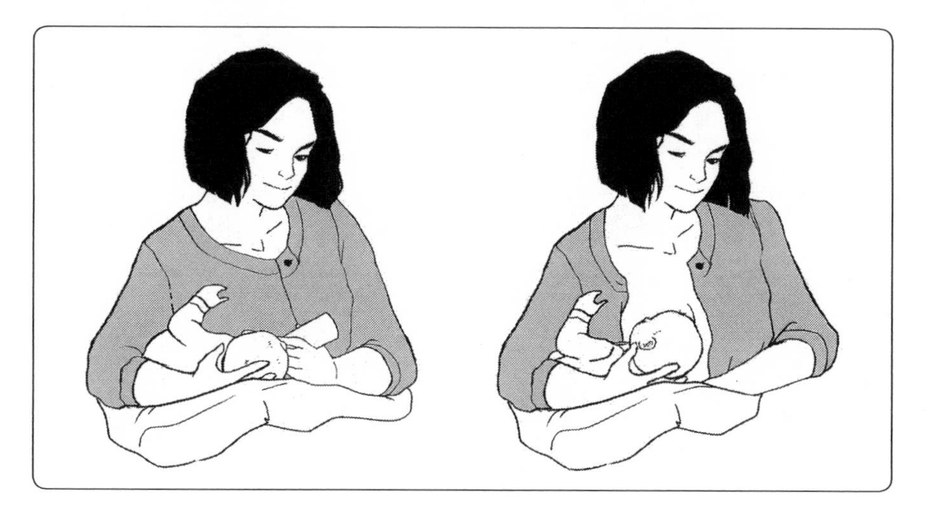

Football hold for bottle feeding and breastfeeding.

The side-lying position works well until your baby's body is too long for your reach. When that happens, you can try the football hold, a position that is often used for breastfeeding. To bottle feed with baby in a football hold, place a long, flat pillow at your side and lay your baby on it in a side-lying position. Ensure their head is above their hips. You can easily watch your baby's face in this position, as shown in the illustration above.

The upright high-cradle position may be tried once your baby becomes a "pro" at bottle feeding. This is the typical position that bigger and older babies feed in. Further details about when and how to transition to the high-cradle position are located later in this chapter under "Bottle feeding."

In addition to trying other positions for feeding, you can also experiment with bundling or swaddling to help feedings. Some babies like to be snug in a receiving blanket, which helps relax them and make them feel safe. Some babies get too hot or too sleepy while swaddled and some like to be bundled from the chest down, leaving their hands free to touch the breast or bottle, or grasp your finger. Some don't like any degree of wrapping while feeding. You and your baby will figure out the preferred amount of bundling.

When to feed

There was a time when parents were told to feed babies on a schedule. Parents would wake up their babies every three hours and make them feed. If babies woke up early with hunger, parents would delay the feed until the set time. Often a feeding battle would develop with parents dictating when and how much to feed. Babies would rebel! Parents would cry! Research has now found that "baby-led," or "demand" feeding is the best strategy to make feedings pleasant, encourage a happy relationship between baby and parents, and to optimize infant growth.

Essentially, with baby-led feeding the parent controls what (breast milk or formula), where (location), and how (strategy) to feed baby. The baby controls when to feed and how much to take in. Feeding a baby involves teamwork!

While your baby was in the hospital, you watched your baby be fed every hour, two hours, and three hours and observed the volumes gradually build from a few drops to a few milliliters to bigger volumes. Now, it may be a bit unnerving to let your baby take control of bottle-feeding volumes. But this is exactly what breastfed babies do. Mothers never know how much their baby takes from the breast. They just feed them when they ask for food.

♥ *We struggled with baby-led feeding. It took us a few months after discharge to let go of the scheduled feeds. I worried constantly that she was hungry... She was most successful at home, in a quiet environment, on a flat pillow, in side-lying position. So, our social schedule revolved around her feeds for a while until she became more successful on the bottle.*

♥ *Most of our worry was about when to feed her. If she wanted to eat again in two hours, I thought, "Oh no, I don't have enough milk," and then if she slept four or five hours, "Oh my goodness, what is going on now?" It's more my stress than hers. She feeds well, but I was so used to feeds every three hours in the NICU. My community nurse gave me a twenty-four-hour volume range and that was the turning point for me. Look at the whole day, not just one feed. This should be taught to all parents before discharge. Maybe we parents wouldn't stress so much then!*

To help you feel more confident as you transition to baby-led feedings, keep a record of your baby's feedings. We offer a simple sample chart that you can do at home. You may find useful apps for such recordings.

Sample feeding record

Time	Breast	Bottle	Wet diaper	Dirty diaper	Comments
	Record time or description	Record volume/ comments			
4:30am	*Lots of swallows* *15 minutes good feed*	*34 ml* *Ate too fast, needed pacing*	✓	*Smear*	*Gassy* *Small spit up* *Uncomfortable after feed. Held upright for 15 minutes then asleep*
6:45 am	*nuzzled a couple minutes only*	*50 ml* *Calm feed*	✓	0	*Gave vitamin with feed*
9:10 am	*22 minutes*	0	✓	*large!!!*	*Satisfied after breastfeed*

Record the details that will help you see a full twenty-four-hour period. You'll notice that your baby feeds at different times and different volumes. This is normal. At the end of twenty-four hours, total the breastfeeding and/or bottle-feeding intake to get a clearer picture of how well your baby fed over that period. You'll see that your baby likely has six to eight wet diapers and some passing of stool. These are good signs that your baby is getting enough to eat.

If you keep this record on a daily basis for a while, you'll be able to compare one day with the next. You might be concerned that your baby does not take in as much on days during which you have appointments or when your baby slept more. But you'll see that your baby will feed more or more often on the following day(s). Your baby's normal output will help you see that your baby is doing well. A drop in feeding along with a drop in wet diapers could be a sign of illness. See chapter 3 for more information on illness and illness prevention.

Once you see steady patterns over time in your baby's feeding record, you can wean yourself off of this recording system. We do not recommend you persist with record-keeping if your baby is feeding and growing well! At some point you need to trust your parental instincts and let go of tracking. But, if your baby becomes unwell, you can return to monitoring what is going in and coming out.

Baby-led feeding helps you and your baby develop a trust relationship. Your baby starts feeling hungry, lets you know with hunger cues, you read the cues, and respond with food. A perfect communication cycle develops.

♥ *At first, I was uber-strict with the feeding schedule and I wasn't enjoying it. I was watching the clock, not my baby. Finally, I tried to feed a little more on demand, so it was every couple of hours and in smaller volumes than what he took before. He stopped throwing up so much. At the end of the day, he took the same or more than he was drinking before and his weight gain was way better.*

Baby-led feeding establishes great rhythm. Your baby learns that you consistently respond to their hunger cues. There is no coaxing or forcing. When your baby grows rapidly and is hungrier, you respond to their cues with more feeding. When your baby needs more from the breast or bottle, you read their cues and give more accordingly.

Parents report that babies develop better sleep routines when they are fed according to their cues. If we wake up our babies to feed them, then their sleep cycles are interrupted. You may notice your baby cluster feeds at certain points of the day and sleeps longer following these. This commonly happens during the evening, at a time when you are tired from a long hard-working day with your baby. However, the pay-off comes when your baby starts sleeping longer at night, usually sometime after six weeks corrected age.

> *My baby was about two months old, chronologically, but only thirty-seven weeks corrected age when she came home. She was so quiet. I always worried that I was going to miss her cues so I set my alarm for every three hours just to check on her. She found her voice around my due date. What a relief that we could finally understand when she was hungry. I didn't need to set my alarm anymore. She became very loud and bossy. She gets louder if I'm slow to respond. I guess that's a good thing!*

During growth spurts, which often happen near term and every month or so, your baby will show hunger cues more frequently. These mean your baby's body needs more nutrition. Respond with a feed as soon as you can. Take naps when your baby does. If you are breastfeeding, keep up your milk supply with good nutrition and fluid intake. Growth spurts do not last long. Typically they resolve after three to seven days.

Identifying hunger cues

Baby-led feeding relies on your baby's ability to communicate hunger. Full-term babies are usually able to communicate hunger shortly after birth. Preterm babies and late preterm babies are often unable to clearly communicate hunger. These babies are still not past your due date and you likely cannot trust that they will wake up when hungry. Premature babies may give very subtle signs, such as licking their lips, or may cue very quietly or for very short periods. These signs are easily missed, but have no fear. Your baby will gradually become stronger and louder. Soon you will not be able to overlook hunger cues. And if you delay responding, your baby will get louder and more upset.

> *She went from zero to starving in two seconds. If you didn't get her when she was a little hungry, it was too late, and she'd be mad. She wouldn't latch on to a breast and she wouldn't take the bottle. She'd just be mad and needed me to calm her down. I learned there is no waiting. She was not patient for food.*

Signs of hunger include licking, rooting, sucking, putting hand to mouth, sucking on fist, being wide awake, moving arms and legs, not settling with soother or cuddling, and crying.

For babies who do not exhibit clear hunger cues yet, a "semi-demand" feeding routine is encouraged. This means that parents do not let their babies sleep longer than a predetermined duration, for example, three or four hours. Your nurse may have given you a suggestion at the time of hospital discharge. At home, you can gradually extend the time between feedings. For example, you start with a maximum of three hours between feeds, and after a couple days or a week, you could try every three and a half hours. That doesn't mean your baby will feed only every three and a half hours. Feed your baby sooner if hunger cues are shown, but don't let them sleep longer than that amount of time. Usually, a full-term newborn will feed every one to three hours, so if your baby cues early, feed them. It is normal for babies to feed at different times. Maintain this semi-demand feeding routine until your baby consistently wakes up independently and demonstrates a positive growth pattern. Remember that the baby is the boss when it comes to when to feed!

Identifying satiation cues

Satiation cues appear later in baby's life than hunger cues. Many babies at term are starting to cue hunger but are not ready to reliably communicate when full, so they may take more and more without giving any cues to stop. Like overfilling your car's gas tank, eventually the extra liquid spills out.

Satiation cues include stopping sucking, a relaxed face and/or relaxed body ("rag doll" arms and legs), closing eyes, turning head to side, and sleeping one to three hours between feeds.

Until your baby is reliably communicating satiation, watch for signs of overfeeding, such as discomfort after feeds, abdominal discomfort, vomiting, reflux, poor sleep, rapid or excessive weight gain. Watch also for signs of underfeeding, including short sleep duration, waking early with hunger signs, low weight gain, crying that stops with feeding. Satiation cues will become clearer when your baby is beyond term. Then your baby will be able to reliably show you when they have taken enough.

Feeding amounts

In our experience of working with parents at home following discharge, the most common question is how much babies should be fed. You too probably feel a little confused and worried about how much to feed your baby at home.

> *When my baby was in the NICU, I watched the painfully slow, sometimes minuscule, increase in feeding volumes. One day my baby was taking 17 ml every two hours, and the next day she could have 20 ml. By the time she was ready to go home, she was breastfeeding a couple of times a day and bottling around 60 ml. I was worried about taking her home because who was going to tell me when to increase her bottles?*

The volume recommendation that the hospital may have given you at the time of discharge is a very short-lived guide. Your baby's needs will change quickly. Watch your baby for signs of hunger, satiation, and comfort after feeds. Consider that the quality of a feed is more important than the quantity. Having pleasant, safe feeds is the goal. Pushing babies to take certain volumes, rather than encouraging babies to feed, makes the feed unpleasant.

A word of caution about advancing too quickly. The size of a full-term baby's stomach is approximately 30 ml (1 oz.). As your baby grows, the stomach capacity will increase, but large volumes might be hard for your baby's stomach to handle.

Variable volumes should be considered as normal. Consider that you do not eat exactly the same amount at each meal. Babies, too, take different amounts at different times, depending on their hunger level. Sometimes they wake up early and want a snack. Sometimes they have a longer sleep and wake up very hungry, wanting a larger feed.

Signs that your baby is taking enough include:

- six or more wet diapers each day;
- bowel movements that are soft, seedy, or loose;
- approximately 140 to 210 grams (5 to 7.4 oz.) of weight gain per week;
- sleeps of one to three hours between feeds;
- positive growth on a growth graph at the nurse or doctor's office.

ACTION PLAN: Cue-Based Feeds

Try these strategies for cue-based feeds:

- Give small, frequent feeds, as they are better tolerated than large, infrequent feeds. Remember that full-term babies feed every one to three hours. Feeding a forty-one-week corrected age baby (one week old) every four hours will mean your baby has to take very large volumes, which may cause stomach upset, reflux, and difficulty sleeping.
- Look at your baby's intake over twenty-four hours, not just at one feed.
- Feed until your baby is satiated.
- Watch for a baby's cues of satiation or feeling full. This is an important guide for feeds. Parents should not override satiation cues or baby will be uncomfortable or vomit after feeds. Overfeeding can contribute to obesity and reflux (see chapter 5 on tummy troubles).
- Don't work harder at the feed than your baby. If this happens, stop the feed. It's time for a rest.

Not taking in enough

When you first took your baby home, you may have noticed that your baby did not feed as well as they did in the hospital. This is very common and seems to be related to a change of environment. It takes a couple of days or weeks for your baby to adjust to the new smells, new lighting, and new sounds of your home. Be patient and feed your baby on cues. Your baby might need a little more comforting and cuddles while settling in.

Feeding is hard work and some babies, for example, babies with jaundice, on oxygen, or with viral cold symptoms (stuffy or runny nose), or premature or late preterm babies, may not have enough energy to take a good feed. These babies may fall asleep after a small feed and appear like they are satiated. It can be hard for parents to know if they are showing signs of satiation or exhaustion.

He was so sleepy and I was afraid he wouldn't gain weight. But I worried that I was burning too many of his calories trying to get it into him, and whether I should be stopping. Sometimes he would gag. I didn't want him to hate feeding.

The doctor said that our baby wasn't gaining enough grams per day. She said, "Feed your baby more." And that was that. No tips or pointers. On the way home, my wife cried in the car. She was exhausted and she was doing the best she could. I was back to work so it was all on her shoulders. She wanted to give up breastfeeding and push bottles. The nurses told us not to push. But we wondered how we'd get our baby to take more.

Our overall key recommendation is to not force feeds. There are lots of things parents can do to encourage their baby's intake.

ACTION PLAN: Increase Intake

Try these strategies to encourage increased intake:

- Feed your baby as soon as they cue hunger. Don't wait till they are overly upset, as they may waste precious energy crying and then be too tired to feed well.
- Ensure your baby does not get too warm while feeding.
- Offer a midway burping and careful diaper change. Some babies get very upset when having their diaper changed so doing this before feeding may make baby too worked up and therefore too upset or tired to feed. After the mid-feed change, they'll be awake enough for the second half of their feed.
- Avoid changing the diaper at the end of the feed, as this may cause your baby to vomit.
- If your baby falls asleep mid-feed, and you've tried a burp break and diaper change, conclude the feeding. Don't force-feed a sleeping baby. Place baby uncovered in their crib or bassinet. Listen and watch for cues to restart the feed. It might take five to thirty minutes.

If you are breastfeeding, it can be hard to trust that your baby is taking enough, because you can't measure how much your baby took from the breast. You can help your baby take more from the breast.

ACTION PLAN: Increase Intake, Breastfeeding

Try these strategies to increase intake while breastfeeding:

- Ensure you have a good supply of breast milk. You should be able to produce more than 500 ml (2 cups)/day. Talk to a lactation consultant, breastfeeding clinic, doctor, or nurse about your supply.
- Ensure your baby has a deep latch on the breast, which will make it easier for your baby to take more milk. Wait till your baby gives you a big open mouth before latching. Avoid letting baby suck your nipple in as this will cause a shallow latch. We cover more breastfeeding latch advice later in this chapter.
- Apply a warm cloth to your breast before breastfeeding to soften the milk ducts.
- During breastfeeding, massage your breast from the periphery toward center.
- During breastfeeding, add compression to your breast with one hand to increase the pressure inside the breast. This will help your baby take more milk.
- Breastfeeding babies can easily get too warm next to your body and fall asleep too early. Undress or unwrap your baby. Take their legs out of the sleeper and tickle their toes.
- Every time you sit down to breastfeed, drink a glass of water. Fluid in helps fluid out.

If you are bottle feeding, it's easy to become focused on the bottle volume and worried when they don't take the full bottle every feeding. Breastfed babies are lucky in that regard, because parents can't see how much they took from the breast. Instead, breastfed babies are fed till they are satiated. Bottle-fed babies should be fed the same way: bottle feed until they are full. They don't need to finish every drop in the bottle.

ACTION PLAN: Increase Intake, Bottle Feeding

Try these strategies to support intake during bottle feeds:

- Ensure the nipple hole is clean, not plugged, and not cracked. Over time, nipples can erode from boiling or sanitizing.
- No matter who's feeding the baby, use the same strategies so that your baby learns to trust the feeding experience.
- Keep the bottle warm. Some babies won't feed as well if the bottle has cooled off. Reheat the bottle if you take a break mid-feed.
- Loosen the nipple collar slightly so that a vacuum is not created inside the bottle when your baby sucks.

Avoid the temptation to get a faster-flow nipple. I tried a faster nipple but he choked after a few sucks. Then I could see that he stopped breathing. So I pulled the nipple and I sat him up and then he had to catch his breath—it just went in too fast. I was terrified. I was all by myself and there were no monitors or nurses.

Newborns need a slow-flow nipple for at least four months. A faster-flow nipple may lead to suck-swallow-breathe incoordination and choking. Find more information on this below.

Waking up baby to feed

Sleepy babies are not good feeders. Waking a baby up to feed is often unpleasant for the baby and frustrating for parents. Babies who wake for feeds on their own will be more enthusiastic and efficient feeders.

If your health care professional advises you to wake your baby to feed due to a health concern, such as low weight gain, here are some gentle strategies to help arouse your baby:

- Turn on a light.
- Play music.
- Uncover your baby.
- Talk to your baby.
- Stroke your baby's face, head, and body.
- Tickle your baby's feet.
- Change your baby's diaper.
- Undress your baby.

A golden rule is not to use the bottle to wake your baby. Wake up your baby's body, not their mouth.

The need to wake your baby for feedings should be a temporary measure until the medical issue is resolved. Afterward, return to cue-based feeding.

What to feed

While your baby was in hospital, you faced the decision whether to provide breast milk or not. Breast milk is the number-one choice for premature babies. Some mothers are able to produce enough and more for their baby, others struggle for every drop, and some cannot produce any. Some mothers choose to provide formula to their newborn.

At home, you need to think about what would be best for your baby's nutrition AND for you. Every mother and family's decision is a personal choice.

Consider:

- If you provided breast milk to your baby in hospital, will you continue to do so at home?
- Is your goal to fully breastfeed?
- Will you breastfeed or give breast milk by bottle?
- Is there a middle-ground plan that works for you? For example, you might plan to provide breast milk for a certain length of time, to partly breastfeed, or to take it one day at a time.

All decisions are the right ones.

It's like being between a rock and a hard place. I knew I couldn't keep pumping forever. But I knew I wanted to stick with it as long as I could. For her. I just couldn't decide when it was right to continue or to stop. Either way, I knew I wasn't going to be happy. It was really tough.

My milk took a while to come in after my daughter was born. I started pumping every three hours right away but was not getting enough. Our NICU nurse told me that I needed to go on medication or I would risk not being able to provide for my baby. I was terrified. The medication helped a bit. Pumping was difficult but I was committed to it. By the time she was about six months old I was no longer producing enough to meet her demand, so we started to supplement with formula. I pumped until her first birthday. I was so proud of myself for sticking with it as long as I did, despite the time and financial strain it caused. (I had to rent a hospital-grade pump.)

There is no doubt that breastfeeding, bottle feeding, and pumping triples your workload. In our experience we highly recommend that you consider what you can feasibly do while still enjoying your baby. Exhausting yourself will not be helpful for anyone. Celebrate the time you're able to provide breast milk. One month, three months, or six? That's wonderful. What a gift you have given your baby.

You heard about the benefits of breast milk while your baby was in hospital.

If you are still deciding about breast milk, here are a few of its advantages:

- Easy to tolerate, easy to digest.
- Saves time.
- Less expensive than formula.
- Contains antibodies to fight infection.
- Reduces risk of chronic lung disease.
- Stimulates vision and brain development.
- Reduces allergies, asthma, ear infections, diarrhea.
- May prevent obesity, SIDS, cancers.

Breastfeeding also helps mothers lose weight and lowers the risk of breast cancer.

Despite your decision to provide breast milk to your baby, some babies need special formula for medical reasons. Some babies need more calories than are available in breast milk. Perhaps your baby's gastrointestinal system is fragile or does not digest properly. Or maybe your baby was born extremely small and needs enhanced nutrition/calories for optimal growth.

At discharge, you would have been told which formula to buy. Be careful as there are a lot of formulas on the market and the labels can be very confusing. Most formulas are made for full-term babies and older babies. There is formula specially made for premature babies, typically those born less than 1,500 grams (3 lbs., 4 oz.). There is formula made for babies who have trouble digesting proteins, so the formula protein is partly or fully broken down for easier digestion. There are formulas made from soy. Confused yet? Buying the wrong formula can really upset your baby's stomach. Take in an empty can or label to ensure you are buying the correct formula. Ask for help in the store.

The hospital staff will have told you how to mix the formula. They may have told you to use the instructions on the can or they may have given you a special recipe. Pay particular attention as to whether you are to use a teaspoon or the scoop from the can to make the recipe. When making formula with water, always use the scoop that was provided in that can. Do not use a scoop from a different kind of formula, as the size may differ. For most recipes, you should lightly scoop up the powder and level it off with a knife. You should not pack or give rounded scoops unless you were instructed to do so by your doctor, dietitian, or nurse.

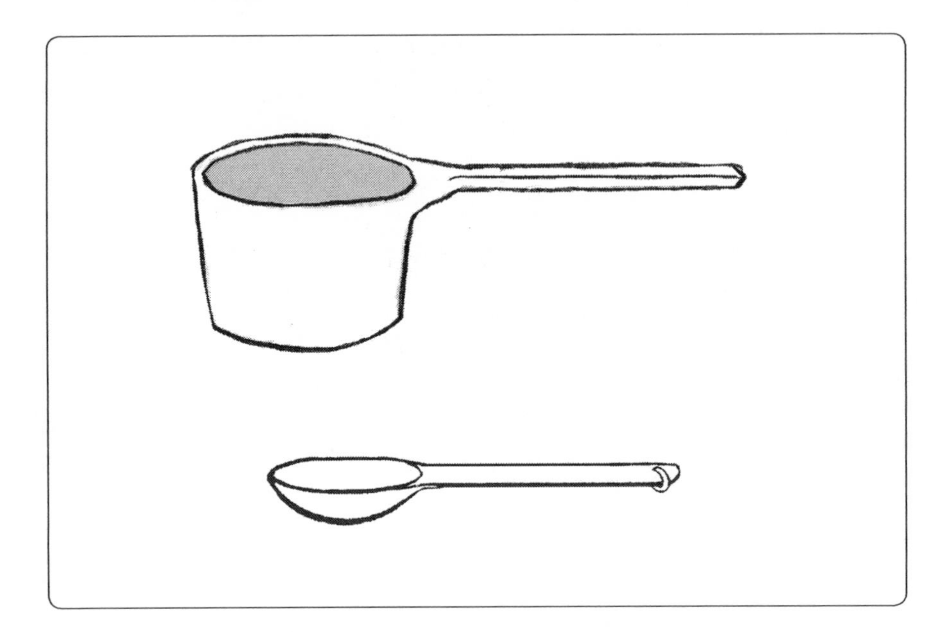

Use the scoop from the can to make formula with water.
Use a measuring teaspoon for fortifying breast milk.

If you are making the formula with water, ensure the water is safely prepared. Follow the instructions the hospital or public health nurse gave you about boiling water. If you use well water, consult your community health department to get your water tested before using it for your baby.

You may be fortifying your breast milk with powdered formula. In this case, you will not be using the scoop from the can. Instead you may be using a teaspoon. Use a measuring teaspoon, not a teaspoon from your cutlery drawer. If you don't have a measuring teaspoon, you can buy an inexpensive one from a dollar store. A common recipe for fortifying breast milk is 1 teaspoon formula powder in 90 or 100 ml (3–3.4 oz.) of expressed breast milk. Again, don't pack or round the teaspoon. Level it off with a knife. Follow the recipe instructions from your health care provider. See illustration above for accurate measuring tools for mixing formula or fortifying breast milk.

Typically, prepared formula or fortified breast milk can stay in your fridge for twenty-four hours. Follow the instructions on the formula can for how long prepared formula can be stored. A time-saving tip for tired, busy parents is to make up a larger quantity of fortified breast milk or formula and place it in a covered container in the fridge, so you don't have to make a fresh bottle every time. When baby is hungry, you just have to pour and heat.

Extra fortification has been shown to enhance weight gain and growth of premature babies. If you are using a special recipe for fortified formula or breast milk, the recipe may need to be changed over time because of high or low weight gain. Your doctor or nurse will guide you on what your baby needs. And, always write down your baby's recipe so you don't forget.

Increasing breast milk fat

More than half of the calories in breast milk comes from fat. You can increase the fat content of your breast milk with the following strategies.

ACTION PLAN: Enriched Breast Milk

Try these strategies for natural enrichment of breast milk:

- Apply a warm cloth to your breast before breastfeeding or pumping.
- During breastfeeding or pumping, apply compression to your breast and massage your breast to enhance breast emptying. Hands on, fat up!

- Pump until you do not see any more milk expressing, and then pump for two minutes longer.
- Pump frequently. Fat content decreases the longer the time between pumping sessions. Regular pumping increases the fat content of your milk.
- When bottle feeding breast milk to your baby, be sure the milk is close to body temperature. Breast milk fat will cling to the sides of the bottle if the milk is cool. Frequently mix the breast milk in the bottle to keep the fat well blended.
- When pumping, stop at the halfway point and change bottles. Feed your baby the milk from the last half of your pumping session. The milk removed at the end of a pumping or breastfeeding session is the richest in calories due to higher fat content. This "hindmilk" can help some babies gain more weight and is easy to digest. Hindmilk is the easiest for your baby because the extra calories come from human milk fat. Freeze the breast milk from the first half of the pumping session to use later when your baby's weight gain has improved.
- If hindmilk does not produce more weight gain, you may have to give fortified breast milk (with formula added) or enhanced-calorie formula (made from a special recipe). High-calorie formula is called "hyperosmolar" and may be challenging for your baby to digest. Breast milk fortified with formula is easier for your baby to digest than enhanced-calorie formula (made from water).

Indicators of successful feeds

Feeding should be satisfying and enjoyable, not stressful. Unfortunately, too many babies and parents struggle with feedings whether they be breastfeeds, bottle feeds, or a combination of both. Sometimes parents miss important messages that their baby is trying to communicate. These cues are important so parents know whether all is well or if a different approach to feeds is required. Examples of these cues are cited in table below.

Feeding signs

Signs feed is going well	Signs feed is not going well
Calm body	Baby is restless, fussy, moving a lot
Relaxed face	Face is stressed, eyes look frightened
Swallowing seen and heard	Arms or legs thrashing about
"Happy yummy" sounds while feeding ("mmm")	Coughing
Baby relaxes during the feed	Choking
Small drops of spillage at lips are okay	Baby arching backward
Falls asleep at end of feeding	Lots of spillage from mouth
Feeding takes 15 to 30 minutes	Color change to pale or blue
Sleeps at least 1 to 3 hours	Feed takes < 15 minutes or > 30 minutes
	Awakens after a short sleep < 1 hour

If you see the signs that feeds are not going well, stop the feeding. Something needs to change. You don't want your baby to learn that feeds are scary or unpleasant. Refer to other sections in this chapter for strategies if feedings are not going well. Keep in mind that if you try something and it doesn't help, it might work at another time. Babies keep changing.

Feeding Strategies

Breastfeeding

If you have been pumping breast milk since you delivered your baby and you plan to continue breastfeeding, first of all, congratulations! Your baby is very fortunate to have this gift of breast milk. If you are not sure what your breastfeeding goals are, refer to the "What to feed" section earlier in this chapter. You have many choices along the continuum from exclusive breastfeeding, to mixed breast feeding and bottle feeding, to bottling breast milk, to exclusive formula. If you are planning to advance breastfeeding, keep reading. If you are planning to pump only, skip to the pumping section.

Practice makes perfect. There is no perfect way to advance breastfeeding. But there is no doubt that without lots of practice, breastfeeding will not happen. Don't wait until your baby reaches a certain age. Don't wait until you get some help in two weeks. Don't offer the breast only once a day. Start practicing now! Even if the practice sessions are only "nuzzling" or "licking and sniffing" for a couple of minutes while the bottle warms. Sit down with the expectation that you are going to practice or play. Celebrate the minute sessions at the beginning and hopefully your baby's practice time will lengthen and become breastfeeding sessions. See the tips in the section "Mixed breast and bottle feeds."

Positions and latching. The two most common positions for breastfeeding are side-lying (also called cross cradle), and football hold (see illustrations of both below). Before you latch your baby using these positions, be sure your body is well supported and that you are not leaning over your baby. You need to be comfortable, so use pillows and foot stools so you can relax in this position.

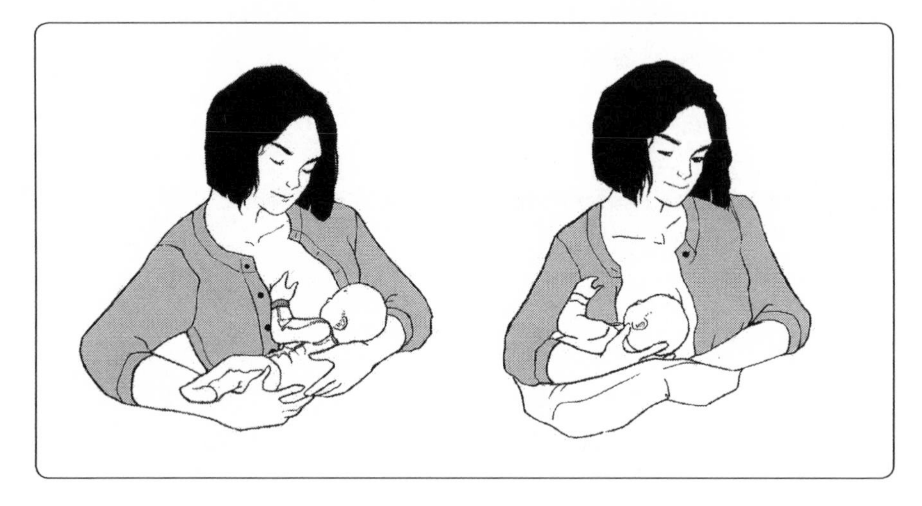

Side-lying and football breastfeeding positions.

To latch in side-lying, position your baby tummy to tummy with you. Use your elbow to hug your baby's lower body close to you and your forearm to support along your baby's back. Your fingers will be close to your baby's shoulders and may gently cup your baby's head (no gripping; this is support only). Your other hand will be used to assist with the latch. Don't push your baby's face into the breast. Baby should be so close to you that they only have to reach up a little to the breast. Some mothers report that they like to position the baby at the breast first, then place the pillow to support baby. See illustrations in the figure above.

To latch while using the football hold, place a long, flat pillow beside your hip. Place a large pillow behind your back for support. Lay your baby faceup on the pillow with head close to the bottom of your breast. If your baby is quite long, you can bend your baby's legs slightly or put another pillow behind your back to move forward. Place an arm to snuggle your baby close to your hip. Your arm will support along your baby's back. Bring your baby's head and upper body up toward your breast. Your baby's head should be higher than the body. Lie back so you are comfortable. Don't lean over your baby or you will get a sore back.

ACTION PLAN: Latching

Try these strategies for latching:

- Encourage your baby to open their mouth widely by gently touching their upper lip with your nipple. Always wait for your baby to widely open their mouth to latch on to your breast. The tongue will then be naturally down in the right position. Wait for the open gape.
- Use one hand to help shape your breast before latching. No pinching or squeezing. Your areola and nipple should be gently shaped between your thumb and forefinger. Keep your fingers well back from the areola (colored area around nipple).
- Let your baby latch asymmetrically. This means your baby will have more of the underside of your areola in their mouth. When latching, your baby's chin should be against your breast and then they reach up a little to latch to the breast. This position puts them in a "sniffing" position with their head slightly tilted back.
- Express a little milk from your breast so your baby gets a taste when latching.
- Bring baby to breast, not breast to baby—when you see an open gape, use your arm to bring baby up to the breast. Don't lean forward to latch. This will put you in an uncomfortable position. Add a pillow under the baby as you like.
- Know that when your baby comes off the breast, your nipple will appear longer and pinker. If your nipple is pinched, white, or has ridges, talk to a health care professional or lactation consultant to correct your baby's latch.
- If your baby is also bottle-feeding, teach everyone to wait for an open gape for bottle feeding, as well. This will teach your baby that a wide-open

mouth is needed before feeding can start. And a wide gape will help your baby latch to the bottle with tongue down.

- Never push your breast, bottle nipple, or nipple shield into your baby's mouth as this will result in a shallow latch and poor milk transfer.

See our website at www.preemiecare.ca for video links on latching.

Once your baby starts to latch deeply, help milk transfer by compressing and massaging your breast during the feed. Be mindful of baby's reaction when you do this.

Easing back on flow. If you're transferring too much milk when you compress and massage your breast during feeding, or if you have a fast letdown reflex, your baby might show signs of "flooding," such as eyes looking frightened, pulling off, spilling, coughing, choking.

For a letdown that's too fast for baby, stop the breastfeed by interrupting the latch with your finger, apply a cloth to your breast to catch the milk spray, and re-latch baby following the letdown. You don't want to pull baby off breast, as that could hurt your nipple. Always break the latch with your finger. It also may help if you lay back when you breastfeed and bring baby up to you with extra pillows. This position helps to reduce the effect of gravity on your letdown reflex. In addition, some mothers need to pump or hand-express some milk prior to breastfeeding. If a fast letdown reflex is still a problem for baby, talk to a health care professional or lactation consultant.

Pumping. Likely your baby did not come home exclusively breastfeeding, so you have been pumping for a while. If you plan to advance breastfeeding or continue providing breast milk, you need to commit to pumping regularly and maintaining your milk supply. At least six times a day, remove as much milk from your breasts as possible by breastfeeding your baby or pumping. One of these pumps should be in the middle of the night when your milk production hormones are the highest. Sorry! We know that's not what you wanted to hear! Regular pumping gives your breasts the message to keep making more milk. If you do not remove milk at least six times a day then your breast milk supply will decrease. If your baby is not a strong breast feeder then you should pump after breastfeeding.

ACTION PLAN: Pumping

Try these strategies to support pumping:

- Pump after baby nuzzles or has a short breastfeed.
- Use a modified sports bra to support pumping. Cut holes in the cups so that you can apply the pump shield to your breasts and thread the tubing through the hole. This is sometimes called a "hands-free" pumping bra.
- Drink a big glass of water during every pumping session.
- Place a warm cloth against your breast before pumping to help open the milk ducts.
- Pump after a warm shower or bath.
- To increase volume and fat content, massage your breasts and then pump. Keep massaging your breasts and pump until the flow slows down. Stop the pump and massage your breast for a couple minutes, especially the areas that might feel full. Try to hand-express some milk. Resume pumping and continue massage. Some mothers report up to 50 percent more milk production when using this technique. Visit our website at www.preemiecare.ca for video recommendations.
- Speak with a lactation consultant or health care professional if pumping is painful or not working well.

Reducing pumping. All mothers rejoice when they realize they don't need to pump as often. Before you reduce the frequency of pumping, be sure your baby is effectively feeding at the breast. Is your baby satiated or needing very little top-up after breastfeeding? If your baby needs a full top-up bottle, don't reduce pumping yet. You could also pump after your baby breastfeeds and compare the volume obtained with the volume you pump when your baby does not breastfeed. If there is a lot less milk pumped after breastfeeding, then you can drop pumping after breastfeeds. Note that this is a simple guide, not an exact science.

♥

By the time you get your baby home, you do not want to pump! You have been pumping for four months. I hated that machine. But if I didn't pump, I'd mess up my supply for her. I asked the nurse how to get off the pump. One way or another I was going to give my baby breast milk. The choice to stop pumping was all mine. I was so done with it. We planned to get going on breastfeeding, and not just twice a day, I mean really work on it. It wasn't easy, but we improved. I nearly kissed the nurse when she said I could pump less.

Your baby should be breastfeeding well at least six times a day before you drop all pumping. Even when baby is breastfeeding six or more times daily, some mothers continue to pump a couple of times a day if their supply is low or if they wish to store additional breast milk, such as for when they are away from baby or need to give extra volume or fortification. Pumping after breastfeeding will give your breast the message to keep making more.

Letting go of the shield. Some babies were introduced to a nipple shield in the NICU. These may benefit mothers who have large nipples and small babies. Nipple shields may also help babies with a weak suck get a longer-lasting latch on the breast. The breast shield should be comfortable for you. Your baby should be able to latch deeply, suck, and draw milk from the breast. You should see breast milk in the shield when you unlatch.

Nipple shields are usually a temporary measure and most babies can be weaned from them over time. Some babies and moms are very attached to the nipple shield and weaning can be a challenge. You can try without a shield when your baby is hungry, when they've had a short feed using the shield, or at the end of a breastfeed. Play with when you try the bare breast and note when baby is more interested in trying. Be patient. This is a new but a more effective way for your baby to feed. Learning takes time.

If you think the nipple shield is too large or too small for you and your baby, or for other assistance, talk to a public health nurse, lactation consultant, or breastfeeding clinic.

Dietary restrictions. Some babies have medical reasons for their mothers to avoid certain foods. The most common dietary restriction for mothers is dairy, such as milk, butter, cheese, yogurt, and also whey and casein. If you are dairy free, talk to a health care professional about what foods to avoid, how to interpret food labels, and how to get enough calcium, protein, and vitamin D.

Other dietary restrictions may include soy, soy products, and shellfish. Mothers report that the two hardest parts of any dietary restriction are interpreting labels and sticking to the restriction. On the other hand, mothers report satisfaction with substitutes for most foods.

Talk to your health care professional for clear advice about what to avoid. A registered dietitian is a very helpful resource.

Seeking professional help. Many mothers and babies benefit from expert breastfeeding advice from public health nurses, lactation consultants, breastfeeding clinics, oral feeding specialists, and doctors. If it hurts or if it's not working, look for some help.

Visit our website at www.preemiecare.ca for links to videos and resources for breastfeeding.

Bottle feeding

Bottle feeding is hard work for premature babies. The suck-swallow-breathe coordination takes time to learn, as does developing the endurance to stay awake throughout every feeding. You might notice that sometimes your baby's skill and energy level are perfect and other times they seem sloppy or tired. There are many ways you can help make this easier for your baby.

Being consistent. Everyone who bottle feeds your baby should do it the same way. Your relatives or friends may have fed dozens of babies, but those strategies might not be suitable for yours. Premature babies need special care and help to learn to safely and effectively bottle feed.

Bottles, nipples, and soothers. Premature babies are more likely to be successful with a straight, narrow neck, and slow-flow nipple, as shown in the illustration below.

A straight nipple means no bumps or sharp angles, just a gradual slope from tip to base. The narrow neck is important as your baby's mouth is still small. As depicted in the illustration below, a wide nipple may result in a shallow latch whereby their small mouth only latches on to the little tip and not the wide part.

This illustration of a narrow latch on a wide nipple shows that the latch is not deep enough and therefore, sucking will be less effective. This non-optimal latch can also be problematic for breastfeeding as the baby will use

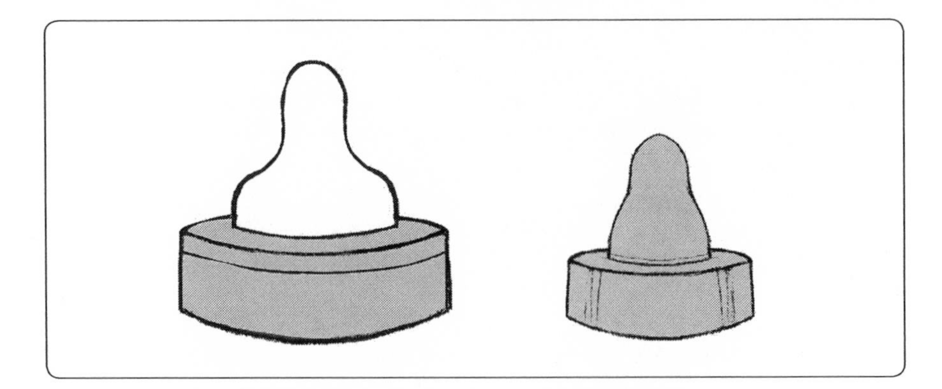

Left: Wide nipple. Right: Straight, narrow neck, slow-flow nipple.

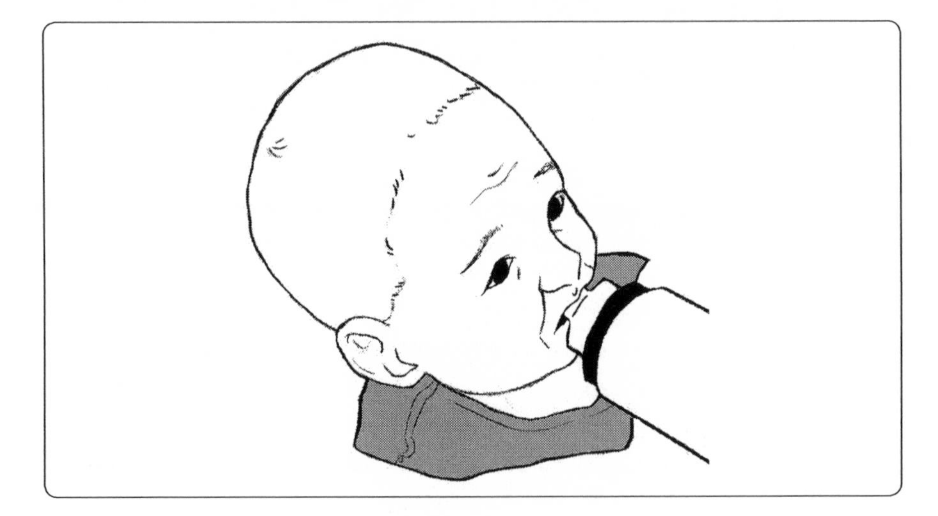

Shallow latch caused by a wide nipple.

this shallow latch on the breast, which will hurt the nipple and poorly transfer milk. Try wider bottles when your baby is older and bigger.

Slow-flow nipples are designed for newborns. These nipples reduce the risk of choking on too much milk, also known as flooding. Flooding is a sign that your baby can neither keep up with milk flow nor breathe properly. Not all slow-flow nipples are the same. There are no commercial standards for what constitutes a slow-flow nipple and some are too fast for newborns. You might need to try a few before finding a suitable flow. A slow-flow nipple is important for babies who are also breastfeeding, in order to avoid flow confusion and bottle preference.

If your baby uses a soother, choose a soother similar in shape to your baby's bottle system. Then your baby will become familiar with this shape and not get confused. You don't want your baby to prefer the soother over the nipple.

Position. Most premature babies need attention to their body position during bottle feeding. We'd like to prevent you from using the most common erroneous bottle-feeding position we see in our practice. We often see babies lying flat on their back with their head turned to the side while bottle feeding. Parents might think this is side-lying, but it certainly is not. Try this test so you can feel what that position would be like: While your head is facing frontward, tip your chin upward very slightly and try swallowing. That is a "normal" swallow. Now try tipping your chin down and swallowing. Much harder, right? And finally, turn your head to the side and try swallowing. That's hard for you and it will be very hard for your baby. Your baby's head must be in line with their body in order to facilitate safe and effective swallows. Also, don't let your baby's chin flex toward their chest. Ensure that your baby's chin is in line with their breastbone and slightly tipped up as in the "sniffing position."

See the description in "Optimal position for feeds" earlier in this chapter, for how to bottle feed your baby in the side-lying position, which is recommended for babies while they learn to breastfeed and to bottle feed. This position will be used for several weeks or months after hospital discharge.

Eventually all babies should be transitioned to the high-cradle position, as illustrated next, which some might call the "normal" position for bottle feeding. There is no rush to transition to this position until your baby is older. The high-cradle position offers older babies the opportunity to combine feedings with a social experience with the person feeding them. Feedings become a time to gaze and interact with one another.

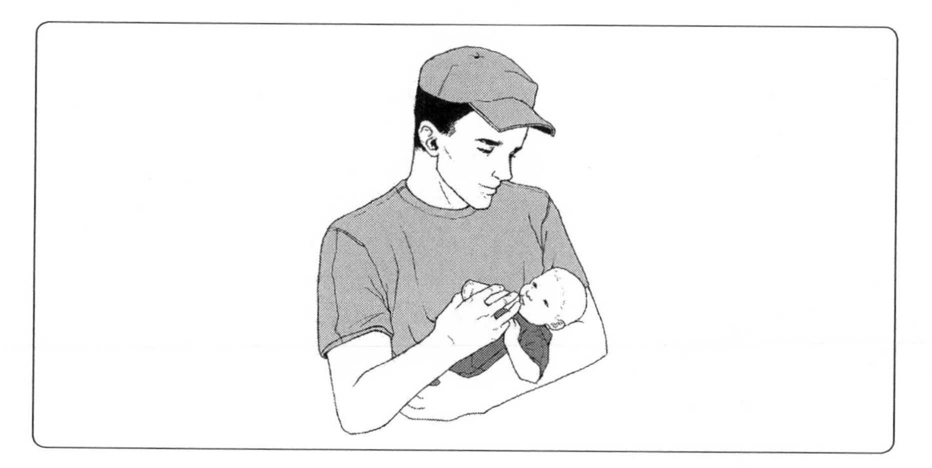

High-cradle position.

Signs that your baby is ready to try high-cradle position include that your baby is:

- not squirming in the side-lying position;
- relaxed while feeding, without any spillage or coughing;
- not breathing fast or heavily during feeding;
- growing well.

To position in high-cradle position, hold the baby in your arms with the back of their head supported in the corner of your elbow. Your baby is leaning back a little, possibly with a pillow behind your elbow and your baby's back for support. Your baby's head should be slightly tilted up, in the same way you would tip up your head to drink from a glass. Be sure their chin is not on their chest as this will make swallowing hard. If your baby shows restlessness, stress, spillage, poor feeding, coughing, or choking, your baby is not ready for high-cradle position yet. Return to side-lying position.

Your baby may be more successful in transitioning to high-cradle position if you try this position after your baby has partially fed in side-lying position and is calmer and not sucking so strongly. You might need to provide more pacing during feeding in the high-cradle position until your baby learns to feed well in this position. More on pacing follows in this chapter.

Bottle-feed latch. One common problem with bottle feeding occurs when we push the nipple into the mouth. The tongue is not in the right position and the upper lip is often curled under as shown in the illustration below. With this shallow latch, the baby's face looks uncomfortable. Lips are pursed together, as though they were sucking from a straw.

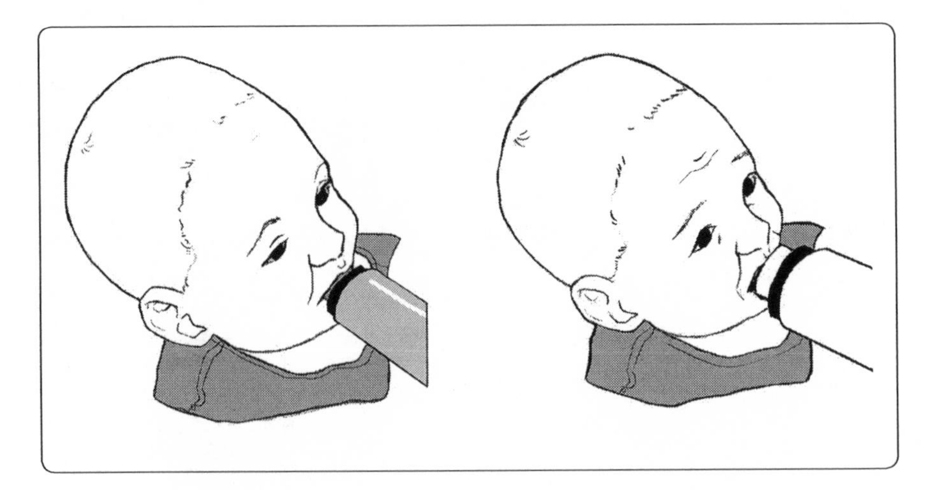

Left: Good latch. Right: Shallow latch.

A suboptimal latch leads to poor suction and sometimes babies will gag if the bottle is pushed in without their open mouth invitation. To fix this, parents should wait for babies to fully open their mouth for the nipple. This is true for bottle-feeding and breastfeeding babies. When your baby offers an open mouth, it's a clear message that they are ready for the nipple.

With a good latch, your baby's face will look relaxed and you should see a little of their pink lips top and bottom. Most of the bottle nipple should be in your baby's mouth. When your baby is bigger, their lips will touch the collar of the nipple.

Holding still. Hold the bottle still while your baby sucks. Do not twist, tap, jiggle, or move the nipple while it is in your baby's mouth. Keep still during sucking and pauses. While feeding, your baby needs to concentrate on sucking, swallowing, and breathing. While paused, your baby is clearing their mouth and breathing. A moving nipple will interfere with these important tasks. If you think your baby has fallen asleep, wake up the body not the mouth. This means rubbing their body, talking to them, sitting them up, or changing their diaper. Don't use the nipple to wake up your baby. Imagine what it would feel like if someone moved a spoon in your mouth when you were falling asleep. This would be very unpleasant and might cause gagging or vomiting.

Too much milk when bottle feeding. There are many reasons why your baby might get too much milk into the mouth and struggle with sucking, swallowing, and breathing:

- Milk releases from the nipple too quickly.
- Some babies have a suck that is stronger than their ability to swallow.
- Some babies have not developed good suck-swallow-breathe coordination.
- Babies naturally suck rapidly on the breast at the beginning of a feed to simulate the let-down reflex. When babies perform this rapid suck on a bottle, their mouths fill with so much milk that they cannot keep up with swallowing and breathing. Babies might choke or become tired very quickly.
- A bottle heated with the nipple attached causes pressure to build up inside the bottle and then milk sprays out when the bottle tips.
- A full bottle tends to flow faster.
- A poor seal between the bottle and nipple collar will cause air to easily enter the bottle and a faster flow.

Below are some tips to avoid excess milk or "flooding" in your baby's mouth while bottle feeding.

ACTION PLAN: Avoiding Flooding

Try these strategies to avoid excess milk in the mouth:

- Use a slow-flow nipple. Try a different brand if your slow-flow nipple generates too much milk in the mouth.
- Use our positioning strategies found in this chapter.
- To prevent pressure build up in bottle, unseal and then reseal the nipple after heating milk.
- Use pacing to control flow and give your baby time to swallow and breathe. (See below.)
- Replace your nipples if flow has increased over time.
- Try a larger bottle.

Pacing for bottle feeds. Babies who present with flooding, or too much milk in the mouth, benefit from "pacing," a technique that provides recovery pauses while feeding.

Pacing is indicated if you see any of these signs of flooding:

- Spillage from mouth.
- Coughing.
- Choking.
- Panicked expression on face, wide open eyes.
- Head and upper body arching back.
- Fussiness or restlessness during feed.
- Frantic or active arms and legs.
- Vomiting after feeds.
- Exhaustion; unable to complete a normal feed.

Flooding is usually caused by your baby sucking in too much milk or too quickly and being unable to keep up with swallowing. Flooding frequently occurs at the beginning of a feed, but can happen in the middle or at the end as well. Flooding is frightening for your baby. It is scary to not be able to breathe. We must react quickly when we see flooding and prevent it from happening in the future. If flooding continues for every feed, your baby will learn to be afraid of feeding.

ACTION PLAN: Pacing

Try these strategies for pacing during bottle feeding:

- Use a slow-flow nipple and side-lying position for bottle feeding.
- Watch for signs that your baby is sucking fast, not taking breaths, or is starting to spill.
- When this happens, remove the nipple from your baby's mouth and rest it on your baby's lip. This allows your baby to swallow the milk and take some recovery breaths. Leave the nipple on the lip so your baby knows it's there.
- When your baby reopens their mouth, place the nipple back in. This invitation from baby might take two to three seconds.
- Upon restarting the feed, watch again for signs that your baby is sucking too fast or not taking breaths. If so, remove the nipple again to give your baby a break.

Sometimes babies need this pacing for a couple of minutes, until they slow down their sucking rate or take short pauses on their own. Some babies need pacing every two to four sucks, some every thirty seconds or so. Some need this throughout their feed, some at the end when they are too tired to keep up suck-swallow-breathe coordination. The extent of pacing completely depends on what your baby needs in order to prevent flooding.

If your baby's recovery breaks are quite long, such as more than thirty seconds, this may indicate that the feed was very tiring and your baby might benefit from more frequent pacing. We see this a lot in our practice. Parents hesitate to remove the nipple because they are worried their baby won't restart feeding. However, the absence of needed pacing will cause your baby to become exhausted and to not finish a reasonable feed. Pace more frequently and note if your baby's recovery is shorter or if volumes increase. Long breaks may also mean that your baby is nearly finished the feed.

The need for pacing will be different for every baby. You might discover that you need to pace more when your baby's suck strengthens. Suck strength normally increases over time, so it's not unusual for flooding to occur well after NICU discharge. We hear parents comment "he didn't do that in the NICU!" Your baby's feeding skill is always maturing and strengthening. With a strong suck, your baby needs a little pacing help from you. As well, when your baby is older, you might find pacing helps them adjust to a faster-flow nipple. Keep this feeding strategy in mind whenever your baby is showing signs of flooding, no matter their age.

Mixed breast and bottle feeds

The combination of breastfeeding and bottle feeding is the most common way to feed premature babies after hospital discharge. Some babies might breastfeed one to two times daily and bottle-feed the rest. Some babies might breastfeed more often but need a small bottle to top up. Mixed feedings create a significant workload. When each feeding consists of a breastfeed, bottle feed, and then a pumping session, there is little time for anything else. Be prepared for several weeks and months of these triple-threat feeds. Unfortunately, that breast pump will be needed for a while. Be sure you have enough support to help you.

All parents wonder about how to progress after going home. To start, you should decide what your breastfeeding goals are and whether they are realistic for your baby. Do you hope to exclusively breastfeed and does your baby's doctor agree that non–fortified breast milk will be sufficient? Do you hope to predominantly breastfeed and give a few fortified bottles? Do you plan to pump and give only breast milk by bottle? All of these decisions will affect how you proceed.

There is no right or wrong way to move ahead with breastfeeding. Sometimes one strategy works and the next day it doesn't. Keep trying or try something new.

Let's assume you breastfed once a day in hospital and explore several different strategies for progressing at home.

ACTION PLAN: Advancing Breastfeeding

Try these strategies for advancing breastfeeding:

- Start out by breastfeeding once a day. When that breastfeed is successful (baby fully takes the feed from the breast), progress to two breastfeeds daily, and so on. This method can take a long time and has a high failure rate on its own, as it doesn't allow enough practice for babies to improve at breastfeeding.
- Offer the breast at each feeding, or most of them. If your baby is vigorous at the breast, let them feed fully. Count that as the breastfeed that day. For the rest of the day, offer the breast for one to five minutes while the bottle is warming. Then offer the bottle and let baby bottle feed till satisfied. When breastfeeding skill is improving, build the number of full breastfeeds. The advantage of this method is that your baby will get lots of practice.
- If your baby already has good breastfeeding skill, breastfeed as often as you like, but limit the feed to a certain length of time—for example, fifteen minutes—then top up with a bottle. Gradually increase the duration of each breastfeed until your baby eventually doesn't want any top-up. Once top-up volumes drop to 10 to 15 ml (less than half an ounce), try without a top-up and assess. Does your baby still have a good sleep afterward? Are they gaining weight and growing well?
- Record the volume of bottle feeds for each twenty-four-hour period. Bottle top-ups should be determined by your baby's cues; thus the volumes will vary with each feed. For example, you might breastfeed and give 300 ml (10 oz.) by bottle each day. Over time, you should see the overall volume decrease as your baby learns to breastfeed more effectively. If your baby is gaining too much weight despite feeding to cues, you can target lower daily bottle volumes. If your baby is not gaining enough, you can work on milk transfer at the breast or increase the daily bottle volumes.
- When your baby needs breast and bottle feeding in the same feed, still try to feed for a maximum of thirty minutes. Feeding longer than this can exhaust premature babies. Exhaustion can affect the baby for many hours.
- Consistently wait for your baby's wide-open mouth for breastfeeding and for bottle feeding. Don't slip in that bottle nipple. A shallow latch on the bottle means your baby might try to keep a shallow latch on the breast.

- Find out when your baby likes to practice breastfeeding. Some babies are too hungry and not patient enough to learn to breastfeed at the beginning of the feed. A small bottle "appetizer" might help curb their appetite, so they can practice breastfeeding. Some babies like to practice breastfeeding at the end of a feed, so they can fall asleep at the breast. Experiment with whether breastfeeding is best as an appetizer, dessert, or comfort after diaper changes or painful procedures, such as vaccinations. Note that babies keep changing their mind about the best time to practice breastfeeding, so keep experimenting!

You don't need permission to progress with breastfeeding. Do what feels right for you and your baby. Use your baby's weight and growth to evaluate your progress. Ask your community health clinic or doctor's office if you can stop in periodically to check your baby's growth.

Troubleshooting feeding challenges

Use the following table to troubleshoot when you encounter feeding challenges.

Feeding challenges

Signs feeding is not going well	Troubleshooting
Baby is restless, fussy, moving a lot Arms or legs thrashing about Face is stressed, eyes look frightened Baby is arching backward Lots of spillage from mouth Coughing Choking	This might be flooding. If these signs occur while bottle feeding, ensure you are using a slow-flow nipple or try another slow-flow brand. Ensure your baby is in an optimal side-lying position, head elevated higher than tummy position. Try pacing every 3–5 sucks to give your baby a chance to swallow. If these signs occur while breastfeeding, unlatch baby from breast, wait until milk ejection reflex has passed and continue. If this persists, mom should try lying back to reduce the impact of gravity on breast milk flow.

Color change to pale or blue	Babies will turn red or purple if they are very upset but will quickly resume normal color after calmed down. If your baby chokes during a feed, stop the feed, lift your baby up to your shoulder, and watch their color. Stay calm and speak calmly to your baby. They should pink up very quickly. If your baby remains pale or blue, call 911. If your baby stops breathing, start rescue breathing and call 911. If there is no heartbeat, start infant CPR. Your baby needs a doctor or emergency department. Babies should never turn blue or stop breathing while feeding.
Feed takes under 15 minutes	Full feeds that take less than 15 minutes are too fast. This may cause tummy cramping after the feed. Is the nipple too fast? Can you add some short breaks during the feed to slow it down? Some older breastfeeding babies become very efficient and may only feed for 10 to 15 minutes. This is normal for older babies who are growing well.
Feed takes over 30 minutes	Feeds that take longer than 30 minutes mean your baby is working too hard. When your baby is hungry, are you responding immediately and not letting them tire from crying? Can you keep your baby awake during the feed by undressing or changing diaper mid-feed? Can you help milk transfer from the breast with massage or compression so your baby takes more? Is the bottle nipple plugged or old? Would your baby benefit from pacing to allow more breaths? Would a break mid-feed help your baby get more energy to finish the feed?
Awakens after a short sleep (< 1 hour)	Your baby may not have fed enough at the last feed. If this repeatedly occurs and your baby is not growing well, follow the ideas about how to help your baby take more from the bottle or breast. If you are bottle feeding, you may start adding more volume to your baby's feeds. Sometimes short sleeps occur during growth spurts. Your baby is growing rapidly and needs more to drink. Just follow your baby's cues for feeding. Growth spurts tend to occur every 1 to 2 months in the first year of life. Their increased hunger will last 3 to 7 days. If you are breastfeeding, growth spurts are also a little reminder to you to ensure your milk supply is optimal. Consider your fluid, nutrition, and rest.

Baby was feeding well, but becomes distracted around 3 months corrected age.	Around 3 months corrected age, your baby will be very interested in looking around and will have trouble concentrating on the feed. Move to a quiet, dimly lit room to help them concentrate. Talk to your baby to keep them engaged. Smile at your baby. Do not chase your baby with the bottle. Keep the bottle in the "usual" position and wait till your baby returns to feed.
Baby was feeding well, but around 3 months corrected age, baby becomes less coordinated or is biting the bottle/breast or pushing out their tongue.	Around 3 months corrected age, your baby loses the newborn sucking reflex. Now they suck because they want to, and not because there is an automatic reflex to suck. This means that your baby has to learn to control their mouth and tongue. It will take a few days for your baby to figure out how to make their mouth work well. Be patient. Don't push feeds. Let them bite, mouth, or chew the bottle. Just keep the bottle still and let them figure this out. Expect them to be sloppy. If breastfeeding, keep offering breast. Sometimes breastfeeding babies refuse the breast for a short period of time, might accept the bottle, and then return to breastfeeding. If you are frustrated, seek advice from a breastfeeding expert.

Preventing feeding aversion

Scary or unpleasant feeds can lead to the development of "feeding aversion" over time. Feeding aversion, also known as oral aversion, results when babies repeatedly experience feedings as negative, stressful, or painful. Babies might have physical reasons for painful feeds, such as gastroesophageal reflux (GER) or a throat problem. Babies might have had ongoing feeding problems, such as flooding or suck-swallow-breathing incoordination. In either case, babies begin to associate feedings as negative. When babies are young, it is easy for parents to misinterpret or miss signals that the feeding is unpleasant. But when babies get older, they will demonstrate their displeasure or stress. They may turn their head away, cry, arch, or refuse to feed. They are hungry but have learned that feeding is unpleasant.

The best strategy is to PREVENT feeding aversion. Watch for signs of feeding stress. If the strategies in this book do not help your baby experience pleasant and safe feeds, please seek professional help. If your baby shows signs of feeding refusal, talk to your baby's doctor.

Reach out for help sooner rather than later. Untreated feeding aversions will involve long-term therapy. You don't want your baby to associate feeding as a negative experience and you don't have to figure this out on your own. Be an advocate for your baby and insist on specialist help. Your community nurse or doctor should provide guidance or help you connect with a lactation consultant, occupational therapist, speech language pathologist, or outpatient clinic that specializes in oral feeding challenges.

Weighing

Your baby was likely weighed every day or two in the NICU. We know that NICU parents relied on frequent weight reports as an indicator of progress!

> ♥ *I didn't realize how dependent I was on those daily weights. When I called or went to the NICU, it was always the first thing I asked. When we went home, I missed that.*

In the first few weeks after hospital discharge, you might want to weigh your baby once or twice a week, just to be sure they are managing their feeds well. Perhaps you could access an infant weight scale in a nearby doctor's office or health clinic. It is not necessary to rent or buy an infant scale. There are other signs that your baby is doing well, such as six to eight wet diapers daily, regular stools, good feeding skills, satiation after feeds, normal sleep patterns for their age, and the absence of signs of illness.

Once your baby is feeding well and has shown good growth, you can extend weights to weekly, biweekly, monthly, or every other month. The frequency depends on your baby's growth pattern. If your baby is feeding and growing well, you don't need to weigh often. You might want to weigh your baby more often (for example, weekly), if your baby's feeding and growth are not ideal, if your baby becomes sick, or if you are making changes (for example, breastfeeding more often, reducing supplements or top-up feedings, or changing formula recipes).

Weight gain

Until about four months corrected age, we recommend weight gain of 20 to 30 grams (0.7 to 1 oz.) per day, or 140 to 210 grams (5 to 7.5 oz.) per week. But every baby is unique. Talk to your baby's doctor about the best weight-gain goal for your baby.

After four months corrected age, your baby will sleep longer at night and be more active. Thus, normal weight gain will be a little lower. We recommend a weight gain of 15 to 20 grams (0.5 to 0.75 oz.) per day, or 450 to 600 grams (16 to 21 oz.) per month at this time.

More important than weight gain, your baby should follow a good growth pattern that can be visualized on a growth record or graph. Your baby's community health care professionals (doctors, nurses, dietitians) will plot your baby on a growth record. For babies under ten weeks corrected age, we recommend the Fenton Growth Chart for boys and girls as these graphs are based on prematurely born babies.

The World Health Organization (WHO) has growth records for zero to thirty-six-month-old boys and girls. Your baby's health care team will likely plot your baby on these WHO graphs. Since your baby was born prematurely, you may notice that their measurements are plotted using their chronologic age (from birth) as well as their corrected age. Where your baby plots according to their corrected age is a better indication of how your baby is doing. Typically, premature babies are plotted on their corrected age for three to five years.

Tube feeding at home

Tube feeding at home is not a common experience for babies and families, but it is necessary for some. It can be the only option to prevent a very long hospitalization, to achieve good weight gain, and to finally take your baby home.

First and foremost, congratulate yourself for taking on this task. It must have been a big decision for you. You have had to overcome the fear of tube insertion and learn how to tube feed your baby. This is not easy for any parent. But you decided to take this on so that you could have your baby at home with you. Your baby is lucky to have you as parent.

You will have learned how to insert gavage tubes, tube feed, and clean the supplies. If you have questions about these, contact your feeding supplier or the outpatient clinic where your baby is assessed.

Here are a few tips about tube feeding at home:

Pesky little fingers. The minute you turn your back, their fingers will grasp the tube and pull. You don't want to have to reinsert that tube any more often than you need to.

Cover their hands and arms with socks rather than baby mitts, which fall off easily. You could also purchase sleepers with material that folds over the hands.

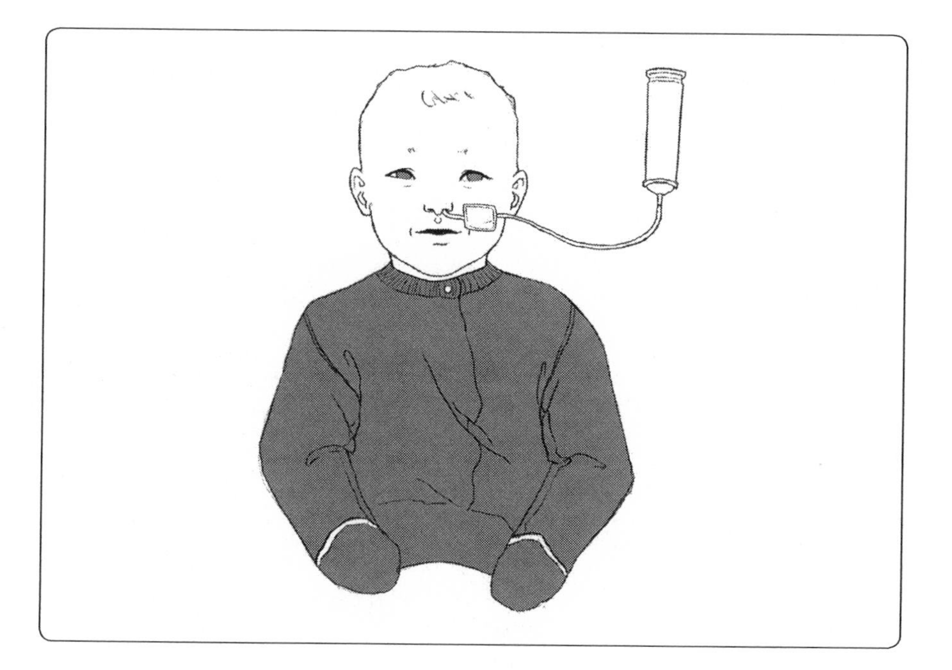

Tube feeding at home.

Parents should also be very proactive at retaping when the tape comes loose. We were often able to retape without removing the tube, which saved our baby and us a lot of stress. When we let the tape fall off, we paid for it later, usually with the tube coming out at an inconvenient time.

To prevent older babies from tubing entanglement, see our suggestions in chapter 3.

Tube feeding is meal time. When your baby is awake during tube feeds, provide your attention (smiling, talking), positive touch (stroking, kissing), and a sucking opportunity (soother). If your baby is allowed to take fluid by mouth, you could add breastfeeding, your pumped breast milk, or drops of milk/formula. Avoid tube feeding your awake baby by hooking up the tubing and walking away. Remember that feeding is social time. Help your baby suck or have a social interaction with you while their stomach is filling to teach them that feeding is a fun time with you.

Vomiting. Sometimes the feeding tubes can cause babies to bring up food from their stomach. Slowing down the tube feed may help. See chapter 5 for more on reflux. Talk to your baby's doctor if this persists.

> ♥ *We found our baby threw up much less when we kept her as stationary as possible during and for a period after feeds. This meant running her feed with her lying on the pillow. At the same time, we would interact with her by reading books and singing songs while giving her a soother.*

Vomiting the tube. If your baby has a big vomit, the feeding tube might also come up. If the tube was inserted through the nose, then part of the tube may be out the nose and part out the mouth. The first time this happens is often shocking for parents. Cut the tube close to the nose and remove both sides. Insert a new tube.

> ♥ *The feeding clinic only gave us three tubes a month, so with our son vomiting up his tube multiple times a day, we had to reuse it. When it came out of his mouth, we would draw it from his nose, leaving the tape intact on his cheek, and then reinsert it. This saved us removing the tape and refastening it, which was a two-person job. Reinserting the tube when it was already taped could be done by one person. The other tricky part was trying to check placement when his stomach was empty. We would reinsert the tube, wait a few minutes for him to calm down, then offer a tiny bit of his bottle. After he drank a bit, we would check placement.*

Feeding hands-free. During gavage feeds, many parents hold the syringe with one hand and baby with the other. This does not leave a hand to help your baby suck on a soother. Ask your feeding tube supplier for a short extension tube with a roller clamp. Then you can use an elastic band to hang the syringe to a pole or hook. Your supplier may also have a feeding bag for when your baby takes larger volumes. This bag and tubing include a roller clamp.

Check a hardware store for temporary, easily removable hooks that can be hung on walls, bookshelves, lamps for hands-free feeding.

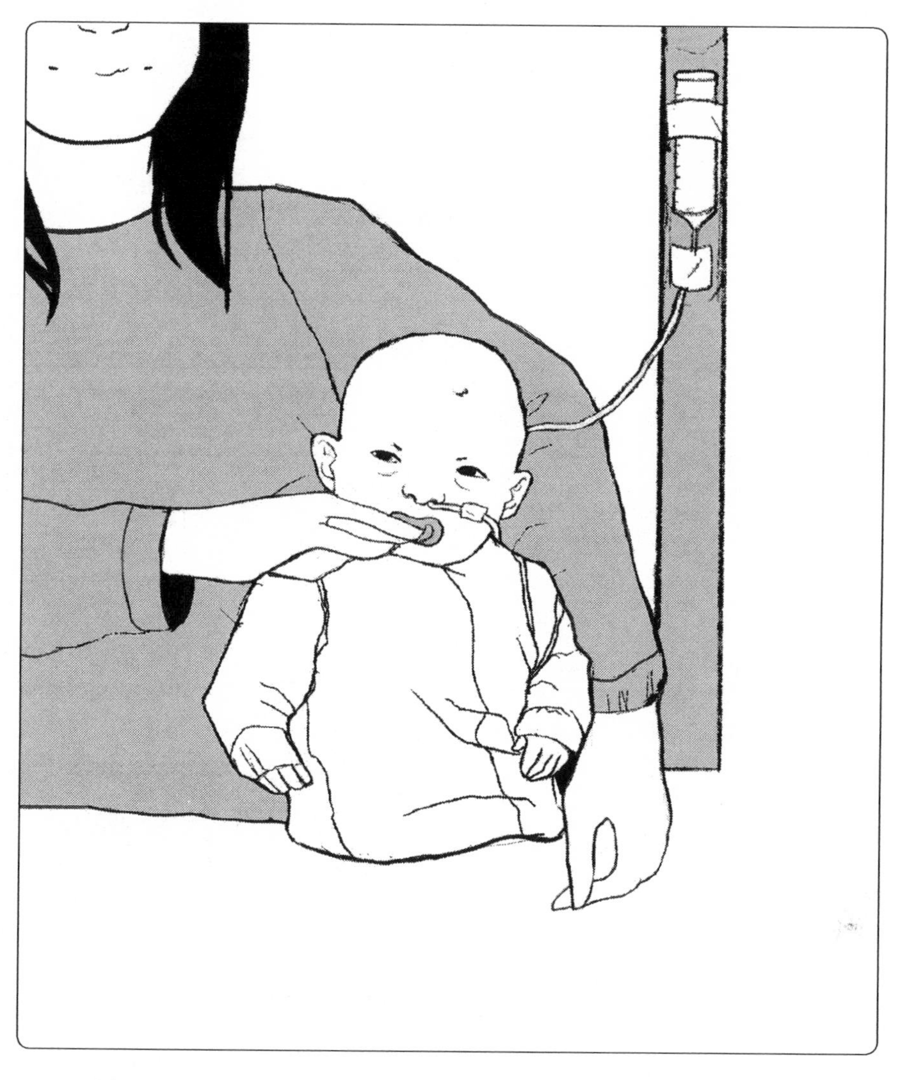

Suspend the feed syringe or bag from a lamp or wall hook to free your hands while feeding.

Setting up multiple feeding areas. Feed in different areas in your home, not just in one room. For your convenience, have several feeding stations, using lamps or other safe fixtures to hang feeding tubes.

Securing helpful resources. Ask your nurse or doctor for a referral to an oral feeding specialist for ideas about positive oral stimulation and strategies for oral progression.

Ask your doctor about an electric feeding pump to deliver the liquid over a set duration. This can free up your hands to work on fun oral play with your baby during a pumped feed. It is tiring to hold up the barrel of the syringe for twenty to thirty minutes. Older babies become more active and need you to have two free hands to keep them contained and entertained during a feed. Your doctor might also suggest a pumped feed over several hours at night while your baby sleeps.

♥ *When you learn how to use the pump at the feeding clinic, make sure to take really detailed notes on how to set the volume and determine the rate, and so on. You will not remember anything once your baby is home.*

Being organized. Leaving the house with a feeding tube can be stressful. Be prepared by having a feeding bag ready for when you have appointments.

♥ *In a large container, pack a couple of syringes (for checking placement and pushing small volumes), some extra tape, and maybe even an extra shirt for yourself if your baby frequently vomits. When it's time to go, throw in your feeding pump and feeding bag, and you're ready.*

♥ *Cleaning tubes can also be time-consuming. After running the tube feed, empty, rinse, and refill the bag. Keep it in a plastic bag or large bowl in the fridge. When you're ready to feed again, warm the bag in a bowl of water.*

Weaning from tube feeds. Weaning from tube feeds is highly dependent on your baby's oral feeding skill. As much as you want the tube to go away, you can't rush the weaning process. Moving too quickly may push your baby to exhaustion or cause them to become fearful of feeds. The process must be baby-led. An oral feeding specialist will be very helpful.

A feeding diary can support the weaning process. The diary should include oral intake (breast, bottle) and tube intake, as well as details about your baby's feeding skills (cues to feed, flooding, refusal). This diary will help specialists (doctor, oral feeding specialist, nurse) gauge how your baby is doing, too.

Consistency is very important in weaning. Learning to feed is easier for your baby when everyone does it the same way.

♥

We made a list of feeding rules (for example, no pressure, feed side-lying on pillow) and taped it on the wall near our feeding areas.

If your baby is also breastfeeding, test weights may be helpful to estimate how much your baby is taking from the breast in order to determine how much to top up by tube. Once you get an idea of average milk transfer, don't do test weights every time as that is too much work for you.

Use the tube less and less as your baby's oral intake increases by breast and/or bottle.

♥

If you see oral intake decrease suddenly, call your occupational therapist, nurse, or doctor for advice. This happened with our baby and it coincided with a period of increased reflux and vomiting, so we needed to rejig our plan to reduce the vomiting and help his oral feeding return to normal.

Once your baby reaches about 80 percent oral and 20 percent tube, talk to your baby's doctor, nurse, or oral feeding specialist about trialing without the tube. Give your baby two to four days to adjust to taking full volumes without the tube.

♥

When we did our tube wean, our doctor told us the minimum volume that our baby needed to take over four days. He squeaked by the first four days, and then squeaked by the next week. By the second week, though, he suddenly started drinking large volumes as the hunger set in. The tube coming out also reduced vomiting significantly, and I realized that the tube was a MAJOR factor in his vomiting. A week post-tube-wean, he stopped throwing up completely (from three large vomits a day to none), and once his vomiting stopped, his feeding skills improved enormously.

The final step of tube weaning took a long time. We were so close—she'd last about four days and then tire out. We'd reinsert the tube and try again the next week. For about a month, we were taking the tube out on Friday night when we were both home and able to watch her over the weekend. Sometimes she'd need the tube by Sunday and sometimes later. Eventually, she got there. Her weight gain wasn't stellar at first, but the doctor said a little loss would be okay as long as she was feeding well and still peeing at least six times a day.

Once your baby is off the tube, feed by infant cues. Offer small, frequent feeds to save energy. Focus on the quality of the feed, not the quantity.

Let your baby explore their world with their mouth. Give them baby-safe toys and let them chew their fingers.

If you feel that your baby is not progressing, talk to your baby's health care team (doctor, oral feeding specialist, nurse).

The feeding tube was our number-one biggest source of stress and anxiety. Many days it felt like we had brought the NICU home with us. Feeding involved recording detailed information, dealing with a feeding pump, rinsing bags and syringes, and trying to prevent a large vomit after a feeding session. The quality of our day was often directly related to how much our baby had taken by bottle. Having a tube-fed baby was very lonely. We didn't know anyone else with a tube-fed baby, and it was hard to explain the stress to other people. On days when he drank very little and the majority of his feed had to go through the tube, we would be profoundly disappointed. Tracking his oral intake helped us to keep everything in perspective and to see a slow improvement (albeit with many ups and downs). When he became completely independent of his feeding tube, it was as though a huge weight had been lifted.

Feeding multiples

What do you need to know about feeding if you have more than one baby? Here is some advice from expert parents of multiples.

- *When one baby wakes up to feed, uncover the other baby so that they can start waking up. Feed one after the other and then go to bed!*
- *My life got a thousand times easier when I was able to feed the babies simultaneously. Experiment with pillow positions and talk to other parents of twins (twin groups on Facebook are super helpful). Once I was able to feed the babies simultaneously, their naps starting to sync and I got more breaks during the day. My general rule was, if you're home alone, feed the babies at the same time. (I used a Twin Z pillow, and when the babies got bigger, I moved to using two Boppy pillows.) If someone is home with you, recruit them to feed a baby so that both babies get nice feeding cuddles. If you can feed only one baby at a time, put the other baby in a fun bouncy chair or play center, or sing to them to keep them occupied.*
- *If you have a big house, buy a small fridge for the upstairs.*
- *Record intake, medicines, and poops. You'll be too tired to remember what's been done and what hasn't. Keep it simple. Buy a plain notebook and make a column for each baby. Instead of recording every wet diaper, I noted dry or poopy diapers (since I knew that I was changing their diaper before every feed).*
- *Tandem breastfeeding can be time saving, but your babies need to be good latchers and good breast feeders first. And, it helps to have someone else there for the first attempts.*
- *Make formula in advance. I gave this job to my husband. I would boil water during the day, and after dinner he would premix the formula for the next day.*
- *If your babies are bottle fed, always have two bottles labeled (if they have different formula) and ready to go in the fridge. When a feed is done, burp the babies and put them down, then go rinse/wash your bottles and make two new bottles. When you have a helper over, they can just go to the fridge for a bottle. Better yet, make a day's worth of bottles!*
- *When one twin is tube fed, offer a bottle to the tube-fed baby, then put the baby on a pillow or bouncy chair near you and run their feed while you feed the other one. Sing songs to entertain both babies.*

Starting solids

Parents frequently ask when to start introducing purees. Solids may be started around six months corrected age, according to the WHO. There is no rush to start earlier. Your baby needs to have a mature gastrointestinal system to digest these new foods and needs to develop a new swallowing skill to take purees from the front of the mouth to the back of the throat to swallow. This happens around six months corrected age. Until then, your breast milk or formula contain all the nutrients your baby needs.

Some babies are challenged when given a spoonful of puree at six months corrected age. A spoon in the mouth, a new flavor, a new texture constitutes a new experience. To help your baby be successful, when your baby is between four and six months corrected age, you can teach them about the feeding spoon in advance of starting solids.

ACTION PLAN: Spoon Feeding

Try these strategies for spoon-feeding practice:

- Buy a small, narrow, baby-safe spoon. Do not use a metal teaspoon that you eat with nor a plastic spoon. Baby-safe spoons are either coated or are made from softer material that baby can bite and chew on. A colorful spoon will be attractive to your baby.
- As shown in the illustration below, sit your baby in a high chair or bouncy chair facing you, so that they can be well supported and relaxed for focus on oral play. Compared with holding your wiggly baby in your lap, a bouncy chair is better, as it keeps your baby's head and face steady. The bouncy chair supports them in a straight and slightly tipped back position. Your baby might need some big rolls placed along their sides to prevent tipping to one side. A high chair that tips back can also be used, perhaps with the same rolls for extra support, as shown below. Many babies are still too small for a high chair.
- Make this playtime lots of fun! Smile, be animated, and make funny sounds.
- Offer the empty spoon at your baby's lip and let your baby lick it, as shown in the illustration below.
- If your baby opens their mouth, let the spoon enter their mouth. Your baby may want to bite, chew, or suck on it.

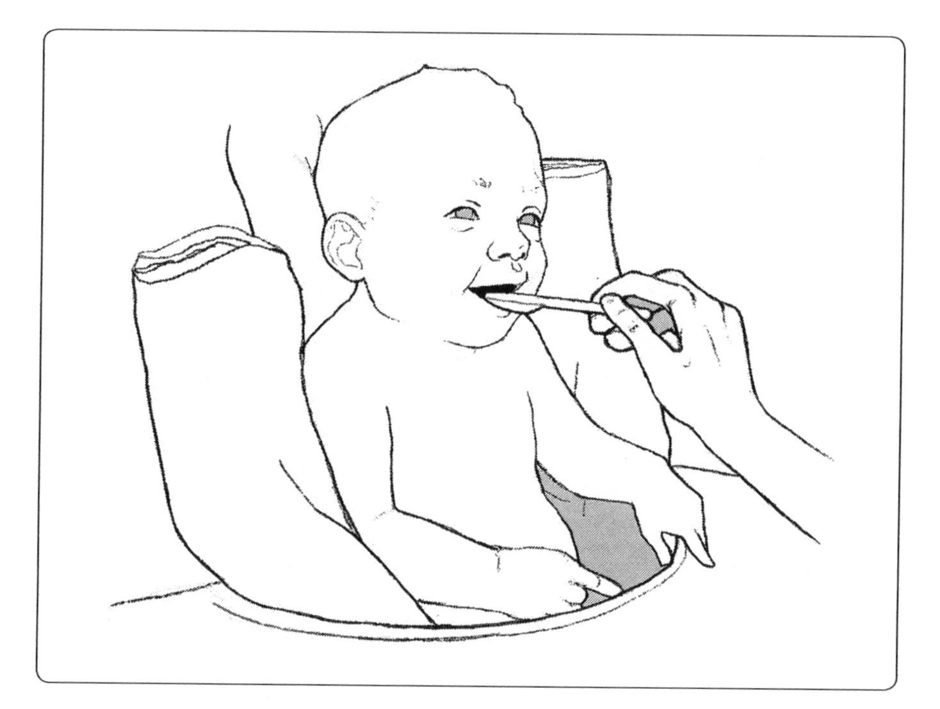

Position for starting solid foods.

- Once your baby regularly invites the spoon into their mouth, put a few drops of breast milk or formula on the spoon. This will get messy so have a bib or cloth ready. It is normal for the liquid to squirt or dribble out of your baby's mouth.
- Keep practicing. When your baby consistently swallows the liquid from a spoon, they have achieved an important skill toward the introduction of solids.
- Include your baby at family mealtimes so that they can watch how everyone puts food in their mouths. Have your baby's spoon readily available so that your baby can join in with drops of breast milk or formula. Don't start other foods yet.

Around six months corrected age, your baby is ready to put new foods on the spoon. What follows are lots of tips for a successful transition to spoon feeding.

ACTION PLAN: Spoon-Feeding Solids

Try these strategies for spoon-feeding solids:

- As recommended by many health care professionals, try rice cereal as the first food. It is easy to digest and can be made into a puree with your breast milk, formula, or water. Don't put rice cereal in your baby's bottle. Cereal should be given by spoon only.
- Start with very small amounts, about a teaspoon once or twice a day.
- Continue to use breast milk or formula as the main source of calories and nutrition for your baby's first year of life. Cereals are low in nutrition and calories.
- Once your baby has accepted rice cereal and has learned how to swallow from a spoon, offer pureed vegetables, fruit, or meat. You can start with any food group, but don't leave meat till the last, as these iron-rich foods are excellent nutrition for your baby.
- Introduce one food at a time. Allow two to three days to assess your baby's response before adding another new food. This allows any allergy or intolerance to appear before you move ahead. Look for signs of tummy ache, diarrhea, rashes, or hives.
- Give individual foods first, before offering mixes. For example, before giving mixed chicken and vegetables, introduce each of the vegetables and the chicken individually.
- Know that as your baby starts purees, their intake of breast milk or formula does not change. Purees are an addition to their diet, not a replacement until they are much older.
- Make homemade pureed food. Steamed vegetables (no salt, no spices, no butter, no oils) make a great meal for your baby. If you have a piece of broccoli or some sliced carrots left over from your supper, mash and freeze these for your baby.
- Use commercial baby food within two to three days of opening the jar, as it does not contain preservatives. If your baby does not like a new food, freeze the leftovers by scooping small portions of it into an ice cube tray. After freezing, place the food cubes in a freezer bag. Thaw and offer this food to your baby later on.

- Allow your baby to play with their food. Place some purees on their tray and let your baby play with the puree and put their hands in their mouth. Remove their upper-body clothing to avoid messy clothes. Clean your baby's face after the meal. Resist the urge to wipe their face during the feed. The more comfortable your baby is with food, the greater the likelihood your baby will progress easily with oral feeding.
- Know that your baby might make a funny face when offered a new taste. This is a normal reaction. If your baby strongly refuses a new food, don't force. Freeze that food and try it again in a week or two. Research shows that babies will usually accept repeatedly offered foods.
- Avoid foods that might make your baby choke. Stay with purees until your baby is around nine months corrected age. You'll notice that your baby has started to chew their food. Now you can start foods with more texture, for example, mashed. Assess whether your baby is chewing and swallowing the thicker food.
- When you move into lumpy foods, watch for choking. Give your baby time to chew.
- Give finger foods for a great eye-hand-mouth coordination exercise for seven- to ten-month-olds (corrected age). Sit your baby up straight in the high chair. Use foods that can be mashed, such as pieces of boiled egg, banana, soft cheese. Do not use foods that could break off into pieces, such as cookies or crackers. Watch for choking. Be sure your baby is able to mash the finger foods well.
- Know that as your baby takes in more solid food, there will be a slowing and thickening of their bowel movements. And they will be smellier! Prevent constipation by introducing fiber-rich foods such as strained prunes, vegetables, and fruits.
- Closer to one year, add food mildly flavored with herbs or seasonings such as oregano, ginger, or cinnamon. Avoid salt.
- Check with your health care professionals about their food recommendations. Your baby might need special consideration if you had a restricted diet while you breastfed or if your baby needed special formula.

Final Thoughts

Feeding is the number-one stressor for families. If you need extra support, reach out to your baby's nurse or doctor and seek help from a lactation consultant, breastfeeding clinic, dietitian, or oral feeding specialist. There is help out there. You don't have to do this alone.

♥ *Feeding after we got home was our biggest hurdle. In the NICU she had great weight gains every day. She was on fortified breast milk and was doing great. We started to nuzzle and introduce her to breastfeeding while on the CPAP and it wasn't that successful. I was stressed. Not only had I never breastfed before, but trying to do it with all the tubes, wires, and CPAP mask, while also watching out for her oxygen saturation level, was too much. Regardless, we tried every day. When she came home, we continued to try breastfeeding once or twice a day. She wasn't latching. We tried a nipple shield; we had a phone consultation and went to multiple appointments with a lactation consultant; and we even had her tongue clipped, as they said she had a tongue tie that could be contributing. All the while I was pumping every three hours around the clock and she was drinking fortified breast milk in her bottle.*

All of a sudden, after being home for about three months, it was as if she completely forgot how to drink from the bottle. She wasn't latching on to the nipple and her daily volumes dropped. With the help of our nurse, we tried troubleshooting everything. I bought a new brand of bottle; we tried different feeding positions, everything. She stopped gaining weight and I was a complete mess. By this time we had also decided to stop breastfeeding in exchange for exclusive pumping. She didn't breastfeed and now she was really struggling with her bottle. I was worried this was oral aversion and I envisioned her requiring a gavage tube for feeding or admission back into the hospital. Luckily, after about a month, she figured it out again.

Starting solids was our saving grace. Our occupational therapist (who had supported us through our woes) was impressed with how well she took to spoon feeding. She has some issues with some textures and was somewhat picky, but I was so happy that we were no longer solely reliant on the bottle for her nutrition. She started to experiment more with solids and is now eating everything that we are. She loves quinoa, cheese, avocado, peppers, and the occasional scoop of ice cream.

We just had her eighteen-month checkup with our pediatrician. She has jumped from the third percentile for her corrected age weight to the twentieth percentile! I almost fell off my chair. Words truly could not describe the relief that lifted off my shoulders when we were given that number. I felt like she was finally out of the woods and clearly thriving. This little muffin has been through so much with respect to feeding and growing and every day we are so unbelievably proud of her.

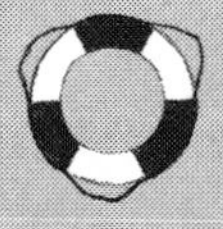

EXPERT TIPS

Here are the key strategies to navigate the journey

- Make feeding pleasurable and safe. You should enjoy feeding your baby. Your baby should enjoy feeding.
- Easy does it. Never force.
- Focus on quality of feeds, not volume.
- Work toward cue-based feedings.
- It's your decision whether you give breast milk, formula, or both.
- If you are breastfeeding, take steps to maintain your supply and practice a lot.
- If you are bottle feeding, use a straight slow-flow nipple.
- Make bottle feeds easier and safer with your baby in a side-lying position.
- Prevent flooding with pacing at bottle or breast.
- Be prepared for oral changes at three months corrected age.
- Weight gain is not the most important sign of good feeding. Low weight gain is just one sign that something needs to be fixed.
- Ask your doctor to show your baby's growth pattern on a graph.
- Start solids after six months corrected age.

5

TURBULENT WATERS
Tummy Troubles

TUMMY TROUBLES are common, especially in the first year home. The premature baby's digestive system is not yet mature enough to work at top efficiency. The gastrointestinal tract, which starts at the mouth and ends at the anus, is not mature until term. In our experience, tummy troubles are a common cause of fussiness, irritability, and crying and a driving force behind frequent trips to the doctor or emergency. Although some problems may need consultation with your baby's doctor, many of these troublesome issues have simple solutions you can try at home.

This chapter addresses those digestive issues that occur in many preemies once home. We cover the most common issues, which include gassiness, colic, infrequent stools, and constipation. We spend a considerable amount of time covering reflux. Reflux is common in preterm babies and can impact feeding, sleeping, weight gain, and growth. We provide research-informed, tried-and-true strategies to manage reflux before resorting to medication. We also acknowledge the challenge parents face when caring for a preemie with reflux.

♥

Feeding and tummy issues were among our biggest issues. Our little guy had already had to overcome so much, it didn't seem fair that eating and digestion were so hard for him. I had trouble believing that it would ever be different. Someone explained to me that there are lots of things that we, as parents, can help move along on the outside but, with the digestive tract, we just have to wait for it to mature. We are about a year past tummy issues, and I can only list about two to three foods our son won't eat. He loves eating and using a fork and a spoon.

Common Tummy Troubles

Gassiness

Gassiness is common in premature babies. Babies have plenty of opportunities to swallow air when they feed, cry, and suck on a pacifier. Many babies do not burp well. Add in the premature digestive tract and there is a good chance your baby will be gassy.

When air gets trapped in your baby's belly, you may notice that your baby:

- burps;
- gets fussy;
- is bloated (tummy is distended, but not hard);
- cries;
- passes gas.

There are many simple strategies you can use at home to help your baby move or expel gas.

ACTION PLAN: Gassiness

Try these strategies for gassiness:

- Prevent gas by burping your baby well after feeds. Try burping baby on your shoulder or seated on your lap. Try patting and making circles on your baby's upper middle back. Tip your baby side to side to work out burps.
- If your baby is asleep and did not burp well, lay down your baby and watch for fussiness. If they become fussy, pick up your baby and try to burp again.
- Gently massage your baby's tummy.

- Pump your baby's legs back and forth (like riding a bicycle) while they are on their back.
- With baby on their back, take hold of their lower legs, bend both knees and briefly apply gentle pressure, moving the knees toward the tummy. The gentle pressure may help move the gas along. Move the knees up and down a few times.
- Place baby on their tummy, but do not leave your baby unsupervised in this position.
- Place baby in a seated position in your arms, with knees and hips bent.
- Apply a warm blanket to the tummy.
- Give baby a warm bath.
- See chapter 4 to read about slowing fast feeders, pacing, and positioning, all of which may help prevent gassiness.
- Talk to your baby's doctor about over-the-counter medications that may aid gas.

Crying or colic?

All babies cry. Colicky babies cry more. Infant colic, or excessive crying in an otherwise healthy and well-fed baby, affects approximately 5 to 19 percent of babies. Infant crying reaches a peak at three to four months corrected age. Colic is defined as crying for more than three hours a day, three days a week, for three weeks. While the name "colic" implies a gastrointestinal cause (tummy trouble), a direct tie between colic and gastrointestinal issues is lacking. Despite much research, the cause of infant colic remains poorly understood and therefore it's difficult to treat.

Often colic is assumed to be related to feeding—something in the milk, the mother's diet, the formula—or to baby's intestinal gas. Recently ties have been made between baby migraines and colic. It is also possible that the immature nervous system of a premature baby makes them more sensitive to stimuli than other babies and they express that sensitivity through excessive crying. However, gastrointestinal issues can play a role in this irritability and crying.

Let's explore ways to determine if your baby's crying is connected to tummy troubles or something else.

ACTION PLAN: Investigating Tummy Trouble

Try these strategies to investigate tummy trouble:

- Try the strategies above to reduce gassiness.
- Experiment with the strategies to reduce crying in chapter 6.
- Rule out sensitivity to something in mother's diet, such as a cow's milk protein allergy. (See later in this chapter.)
- Talk to your baby's doctor about formula tolerance.
- Monitor your baby for constipation.
- Try our conservative reflux strategies. (See later in this chapter.)
- Look into food allergies if your baby is spoon feeding.
- Discuss probiotics with your baby's doctor. Some parents note some improvement in their premature baby's comfort and crying.

Colic can cause parent or caregiver frustration, especially when they are also tired. Excessive crying has also been linked with shaken baby syndrome, which is a brain injury sustained by a baby who has been shaken. Shaking your baby can cause serious, irreversible brain damage or even death. Therefore, it is most important to equip yourself with a tool kit of strategies to manage a baby who has excessive and inconsolable crying. Please refer to chapter 6 for strategies on temperament and crying, and chapter 7 for looking after yourself.

♥ *A month after coming home our son developed colic. It was like he was two different babies. During the day, he ate without difficulty, slept well, and never fussed. But every evening at 7 p.m. it was like a flip switched. He would cry inconsolably until 10 or 11 p.m. and then it would just subside.*

We tried everything: over-the-counter medications for colic, hypoallergenic formulas, and reflux medication. Nothing worked. My husband used to drive him around in the car. We tried putting him in the car seat on the dryer hoping the vibration would work, but he cried. We tried swings and bouncy chairs, but he still cried. The only solution was to take turns walking him around the house at a particular pace.

His colic was one of the hardest things to deal with in our first year at home. We felt so bad as parents, knowing our baby was in distress and all we could do was bide our time and walk in circles. Eventually, when he was about four months corrected age, it just stopped.

Infrequent stools

Infrequent passing of stool is very common in premature babies. Babies may not produce stool every day, but when they do it should be of a soft consistency. Most babies do not have an exact pattern for stool; sometimes they poop several times a day, and sometimes they go days without. They may grunt, strain, and be gassy in the days between stools. These babies continue to feed and sleep normally. This is not constipation.

Having infrequent bowel movements often resolves as your baby's tummy matures and functions more regularly. Sometimes it's just a matter of time and your baby will naturally have a normal, soft stool. But if your baby is fussy and straining, and if having infrequent stools is interfering with feeding and sleep, parents will want to know how to help. Let's consider some options.

ACTION PLAN: Infrequent Stools

Try these strategies if infrequent stools are problematic for your baby:

- Increase breast milk intake, if possible.
- Ensure that you mix formula correctly. (See chapter 4, "What to feed" for instructions on mixing formula.)
- Check that your baby is having the normal number of wet diapers. Low intake or dehydration can be a cause of infrequent stools. (See our "Strategies for dehydration" in chapter 3.)
- Try the above strategies for relieving gas.

- Speak to your baby's doctor about offering prune juice or nectar (this may not be appropriate for babies with history of tummy troubles, such as necrotizing enterocolitis [NEC] or bowel surgery). Although your baby is not constipated, a little prune nectar can increase bowel motility. Most babies respond to very small amounts of prune nectar, for example 5 to 10 ml (1 to 2 tsp) each morning. Your doctor will advise about a suitable amount for your baby's weight. For babies less than six months corrected age, be sure to use pure prune nectar or prune juice with no additional juices. After six months corrected age, strained prunes and whole-grain infant cereals may be given to your baby to aid infrequent stooling.

♥ *I remember, so clearly, sitting up at 3 a.m. and googling disorders that cause infrequent stools. He was so gassy and uncomfortable, but he would go a week and a half without pooping! We tried everything and nothing seemed overly effective. When he hit between four and five months corrected age, it just changed, and he started going daily. He is seventeen months corrected now and I must remind myself of those times, when I sigh while changing my fourth dirty diaper of the day. It is hard to believe that it will ever get better, but it usually does.*

Constipation

Constipation is the infrequent passage of painful and hard stools, or excessive straining during bowel movements. A baby's bowel movements are typically soft, which makes them easy to pass. Constipation is rare if your baby consumes only breast milk. Breast milk is well absorbed and very little remains in the bowel after digestion. Some breastfed babies have several small movements or "smears" throughout the day. It is not unusual for breastfed babies to pass stool every four to five days or more. If a breastfed baby is not straining, uncomfortable, or irritable, it is fine to go seven or more days between bowel movements. A formula-fed baby typically has one to two bowel movements a day for the first couple months and then slows down to every two to three days.

Many additional factors influence a premature baby's bowel and can lead to constipation. Weaker tummy muscles make it difficult to pass stool while also relaxing the muscles around the rectum. Gut motility may be slower in a premature baby. Illness, stress, and medications may also slow the bowels. In addition, many preterm babies are not solely breastfed and often require fortification with extra calories from formula. These formulas are not as well digested as breast milk, so there is more stool and it is thicker. All these factors can lead to constipation.

When cereal and other solids are introduced, this may slow the bowels even further. Low fiber intake will lead to constipation. Switching from breast milk to cow's milk also commonly causes constipation. Do not introduce whole milk until after twelve months corrected age.

Regular bowel movements are important to your baby's health. Bowel habits—how often, how much, and so on—will vary from baby to baby. Some go more than once a day; others will skip a day. You will get to know your baby's routine. If bowel movements are soft and easily passed, there is no cause for concern.

Signs of constipation include:

- stool that is hard, dry, or pellet-like;
- straining, grunting, pushing, restlessness, fussiness;
- not sleeping as well;
- discomfort or pain;
- full, rounded or firm tummy;
- taking longer than ten minutes to pass a stool;
- eating reduced volumes.

Treatment for constipation depends on your baby's age and other contributing factors. Consider the following suggestions.

ACTION PLAN: Constipation

Try these strategies for constipation:

- Look for signs that your baby is dehydrated. (See "Strategies for dehydration" in chapter 3.)
- Increase breast milk intake, if possible.
- Ensure that you mix formula correctly. (See chapter 4, "What to feed" on for instructions on mixing formula.)
- Try the above action plan for gassiness as these provide effective tummy support during bowel movements.

- For babies under six months corrected age, speak to your baby's doctor about offering pure prune juice or nectar. Babies with a history of tummy issues (NEC, bowel surgery, allergic colitis, blood in stool) should not start prune juice without a doctor's recommendation. Most babies with constipation respond to small amounts of prune nectar, for example 10 to 20 ml (2 to 4 tsp) each morning. Your doctor will advise a suitable amount for your baby's weight.
- For babies under six months corrected age, talk to your doctor before using glycerin suppositories. Suppositories are usually not recommended as they can be habit-forming and are typically used only for rectal disimpaction or clearing hard, dry stool from the rectum.
- For infants over six months corrected age, offer sorbitol-containing fruits and fruit juices. Prunes are our top recommendation.
- For infants over six months corrected age, give higher-fiber foods, such as fruits, vegetables, and barley cereal. These foods relieve constipation because their fiber draws water into the bowel to soften the stool.
- If the above strategies are ineffective, talk to your doctor about whether medications are recommended. Lactulose is effective in normalizing stools in 90 percent of babies within two weeks. Always discuss any treatments with your baby's health care provider before starting.

Diarrhea

Diarrhea is more frequent bowel movements than normal with stool that is watery and often explosive. There are many causes of diarrhea, most often a virus. A common cause of acute infectious diarrhea is rotavirus. The germs that cause diarrhea spread easily. You can reduce the spread of the virus by washing your hands carefully after every diaper change, after going to the toilet, and before preparing and eating food.

Babies with diarrhea can lose fluids quickly. Diarrhea can be dangerous if not managed properly because it drains water and electrolytes from your baby's body. If these fluids are not replaced quickly, your baby can become dehydrated and may need to be hospitalized. If you see signs of dehydration, as listed in "Strategies for dehydration" in chapter 3, contact your baby's doctor or seek medical advice at a local clinic or hospital.

You can prevent severe diarrhea caused by rotavirus by having your baby vaccinated. Most rotavirus vaccination programs have a maximum age limit for the first dose, such as before fifteen weeks of age. Ask a community health nurse or doctor about the specific details in your area.

ACTION PLAN: Diarrhea

Try these strategies for diarrhea:

- Monitor how frequently diarrhea is occurring.
- Look for other signs of illness, such as low urine output or fever.
- Wash your hands very well and frequently. These viruses are spread by direct contact. Change the bathroom towel frequently or use paper towel to dry your hands. Do not touch the taps with your clean hands.
- Use a barrier cream or ointment on your baby's bottom to prevent skin irritation.
- If you are breastfeeding, keep doing so on demand.
- If you are formula feeding, continue feeding formula as usual. Do not dilute the formula.
- If you are giving breast milk and formula, try giving only breast milk or increasing the amount of breast milk, if possible. Breast milk is very healing to a baby's gut.
- If diarrhea persists, if your baby is not drinking well, or if your baby has dry diapers for six hours, seek medical advice from a doctor.

Vomiting

Vomiting is the forceful throwing up of large amounts from the stomach to the mouth. Healthy babies will occasionally vomit after a feed. Sometimes this happens when a baby coughs or drank too fast. Before assuming your baby is sick, rule out other causes. Consider what happened just before the vomit. Did baby overfeed? Was baby moved right after a feed? Was baby choking on some milk and so threw up? Did baby have a big burp and accidentally bring up the whole feed? Was baby straining for a bowel movement? These are common causes of a baby's vomiting and do not indicate sickness. If the answer to any of these questions is yes, simply feed your baby again when your baby cues interest in feeding.

Calm baby after vomiting and then monitor for other signs of illness, such as a high or low temperature or diarrhea. See the action plans for high/low temperature and dehydration in chapter 3. If the vomiting repeats or if your baby shows other signs of illness, seek medical advice from a doctor. Follow handwashing instructions as outlined in chapter 3.

Spitting up

Spitting up is the effortless bringing up of small amounts from the stomach to the mouth. Many babies spit up regularly and are not uncomfortable or in pain. A normal volume is approximately one to three mouthfuls. Spit-ups commonly occur right after a feed with a burp or dribble out of the mouth. Spitting up should not affect feeding, sleeping, weight gain, or growth. Babies who spit up normally give clear hunger cues, feed well, and are comfortable after feeds. They are sometimes called "happy spitters." Usually no parent action is required, however you can try some strategies to minimize the effects of spit-up.

ACTION PLAN: Happy Spitters

Try these strategies for happy spitters:

- Hold your baby upright after feeds.
- Burp your baby on your shoulder. Avoid bending them forward and squishing their tummy.
- Burp well and often.
- Increase breast milk intake.
- Give smaller and more frequent feeds.
- Keep their neck skin clean. A bib might help protect their clothes. A burp cloth is recommended for you to protect your clothes.
- You may also try strategies listed in the section on reflux that follows.

Reflux and Milk Allergies

Reflux

Gastroesophageal reflux (GER) also known as reflux is when stomach contents (food and stomach acid) move into the esophagus (the tube that carries food from the mouth to the stomach). Reflux can happen when a baby burps, moves, hiccups, coughs, sneezes, strains, or has a bowel movement. It often happens when a baby is active. Reflux is seen most often in the first nine months and usually goes away by the time babies are one year old.

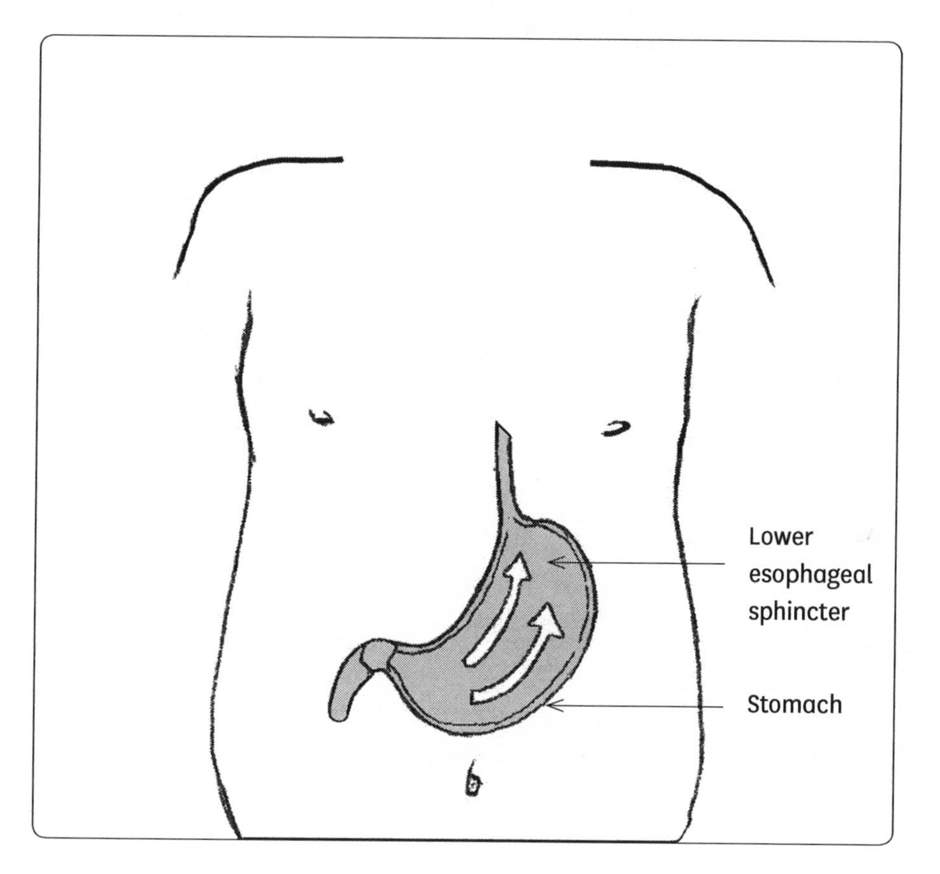

Reflux physiology.

Reflux is more common in babies born prematurely. Usually, the muscular band that surrounds the esophagus at the entry to the stomach (called the lower esophageal sphincter or LES) contracts or closes, keeping the stomach contents in the stomach. In premature babies, this muscular band is immature and does not close properly. This problem can develop in the NICU, can continue at home, or can develop after discharge from hospital.

> *We noticed some signs of reflux before we left the NICU, but our son's volumes were so low we didn't see all the symptoms until we were home. Reflux became more obvious when his volumes increased. Life became more complicated, as we didn't have the time to hold him up for an hour after feeds. We had lots of appointments and had to drive our four-year-old to and from preschool. The car seat made my son throw up more. Reflux made life stressful. I would panic every time I heard him cough.*

Gastroesophageal reflux (GER) may be simple, invisible, or severe, as described in the table below. GER or simple reflux is usually visible and involves moderate or large amounts of vomit that may be projectile.

Reflux may also be invisible. Invisible reflux (or "silent" or "hidden" reflux) involves little or no apparent vomiting. Your baby is still experiencing the upward movement of stomach contents causing pain and injury from acidic stomach contents. If your baby has symptoms of reflux, but does not vomit, it is still important for you to start our anti-reflux actions. Although your baby is not vomiting, the symptoms indicate your baby is in pain and needs your help to manage the reflux symptoms.

Severe reflux may be called gastroesophageal reflux disease (GERD). GERD is associated with problems with feeding, weight gain, growth, and sleep. The acidic stomach contents have irritated the sensitive lining of the esophagus and caused injury and pain. The pain can feel like heartburn. If the reflux is not treated, your baby comes to learn that feeding is associated with pain. This can lead to feeding refusal and long-term feeding problems as babies adopt behaviors to avoid it. See "Preventing feeding aversion" section in chapter 4.

Signs of reflux

	Simple Reflux (GER)	Hidden Reflux (Silent or Hidden)	Severe Reflux (GERD)
Vomiting	Vomiting sometimes projectile or forceful No discomfort or pain	No vomiting but may gag or retch Dry swallows happen when baby feels the milk coming up the back of their throat Face may turn red and eyes may water May have a worried look or grimace Sour milk breath	Vomiting often projectile or forceful Gagging or choking Face may turn red and eyes may water May have a worried look or grimace Sour milk breath
Feeding	Clear hunger cues Feeds well	May only feed when asleep Fussy, arches/squirms or is irritable during and after feeds Coughs or gags during or after feeds Feeds may take a long time Shows signs of hunger but won't feed or only feeds small amounts Seems in discomfort and pain	May only feed when asleep Fussy, arches/squirms or is irritable during and after feeds Coughs or gags during or after feeds Feeds may take a long time Shows signs of hunger but won't feed or only feeds small amounts Seems in discomfort or pain
Weight Gain	Good weight gain and growth	May not gain weight as well	Poor weight gain and growth
Sleep	Normal sleep pattern	Restless sleep Wakes with a painful cry or cough	Restless sleep Wakes with a painful cry or cough

Go to the hospital immediately if your baby has problems breathing, has repeated large, forceful vomiting, refuses to drink for more than six hours, has vomit that is bright green, brown, or black (looks like coffee grounds).

Before you assume your baby has reflux, rule out other factors that can cause reflux-like symptoms:

- **Incorrect mixing of formula or fortified breast milk.** Double-check the recipe for formula or breast milk fortification. If mixed incorrectly, the concentration can affect digestion and cause an increase in vomiting or spit-ups.
- **Exposing the baby to secondhand smoke.** Avoid exposure to secondhand smoke as research shows this can increase coughing and result in reflux.
- **Baby is sick.** Check for symptoms of illness, as your baby may experience more reflux when they're not feeling well. When coughing, it is particularly hard for babies to keep their food in their stomach.
- **Overfeeding or forced feeding.** This is a common and easily correctable cause of reflux. Using moderately smaller-volume feedings and respecting your baby's feeding cues can help reduce reflux. If your baby is gaining excessive amounts of weight, this may indicate that you are overfeeding.
- **Poor or uncoordinated feeding skills.** Suck-swallow-breathing incoordination is common in preterm babies. Rapid feeding, swallowing air, and gulping can produce reflux-like symptoms. See chapter 4 for tips on managing flow, pacing feeds, and positioning for improved suck-swallow-breathing coordination and reduction in reflux symptoms.
- **Excessive crying.** Crying babies may swallow air and this may lead to reflux symptoms. See chapter 6 for ways to reduce crying and settle a crying baby.
- **Straining.** Straining due to infrequent stools or constipation may cause symptoms of reflux. Refer to the above action plans for managing infrequent passing of stool or constipation.
- **Allergy to cow's milk protein.** An allergy to cow's milk protein causes delayed stomach emptying, poor bowel motility, and vomiting. See section later in this chapter on this topic.

If the above factors do not apply to your baby, follow our strategies for reflux.

Strategies to address reflux

Many strategies can reduce reflux. The objective is to do whatever is possible to keep the food down, while making it easier for your baby's digestive system to move food from the stomach to the intestines. The strategies below may be called "conservative" or "first-line" strategies, which are designed for parents to try and then monitor baby for a change in reflux. In our experience, these are the easiest and simplest strategies that can make a difference. These strategies have been shown to decrease reflux symptoms in up to 50 percent of babies and resolve symptoms in up to 25 percent of babies.

In our experience, these strategies, rather than medication, are the best place to start in managing reflux. Why add a medication when something else may do the trick? We have seen babies benefit greatly from these techniques and, in fact, we often suggest them for babies who don't have reflux symptoms. Promotion of stomach comfort and digestion are appreciated by all premature babies! Give these strategies a try.

Breast milk is best. Breast milk is easy to digest because it has digestive enzymes and quickly empties from the stomach.

Feed at a moderate pace. Babies who feed too quickly are more likely to have reflux. Make sure you are using the correct nipple for your baby's age and sucking ability. A nipple that is too fast will fill your baby's stomach too quickly and may cause reflux. Also, if your baby feeds in less than fifteen minutes, give your baby a break halfway through the feed. Burp your baby more often to slow down the feeding time to twenty to thirty minutes. This short break lets the stomach empty a little.

Give small feedings more often. Large feedings can make your baby uncomfortable and increase reflux. It is normal for a term baby to feed in small amounts every one to three hours. This is much more comfortable for a baby's stomach. Compare reflux and how comfortable your baby is after a large feed versus a smaller feed.

Don't overfeed. Watch for signs your baby is full (relaxed body, sleeping). If you try to make your baby drink more, they may throw up. If your baby does vomit, give your baby a feeding break and feed again when your baby shows hunger cues.

Hold baby upright for bottle feeding. Some babies prefer a raised side-lying position. In all positions, your baby's head should be higher than their legs.

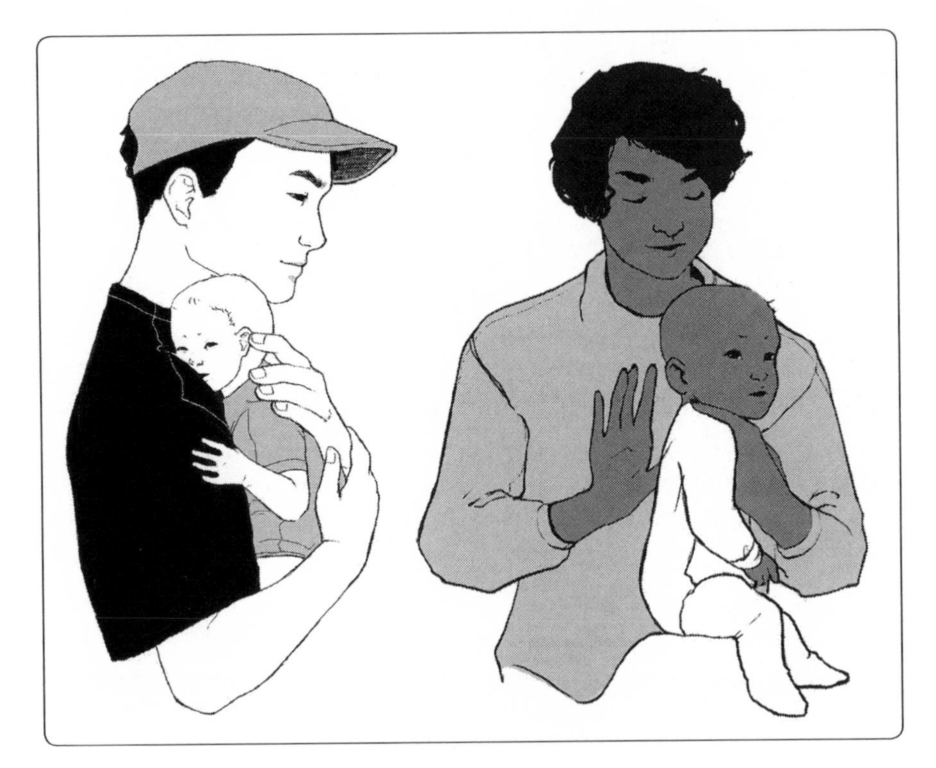

Burping positions for babies with reflux.

Handle your baby gently after feedings. Avoid active play, changing diaper or clothes, or buckling into a car safety seat right after a feed.

Burp your baby. Do so every five to ten minutes while breastfeeding. If bottle feeding, burp your baby every 30 to 60 ml (1 to 2 oz.). Burp on the shoulder, as shown above. This is better for some babies than being in a bent-over position. Watch your baby's face to monitor for spit-up or choking. You can also burp your baby seated upright on your lap as shown above. Do not bend your baby over too far as this can put pressure on the abdomen and may make your baby vomit.

Keep your baby upright after feeds. This will help keep food in the stomach. The best position is holding your baby up against your chest. When your baby is bent forward or slouched, pressure on the stomach may push food up and cause reflux. This should be done for approximately twenty minutes following a feed. Try using a baby reclining seat or "bouncy" chair if you can't hold your baby for that long. Do not use the car seat for this.

Carry baby in a front pack. This will keep baby upright and straight. "Sling" carriers bend your baby's body too much and may cause reflux.

Avoid car seats after feedings. Sitting in a car seat may put pressure on your baby's stomach and cause reflux. Do not give your baby a full feed before buckling into the car seat; feed partially and continue the feed once out of the car seat. When you reach your destination, remove your baby from the car seat. Only use a car seat when traveling in a vehicle.

Prevent baby from sliding into crooked positions. Keep your baby's head and body straight and centered when they are sitting in a bouncy chair, swing, or stroller. Place a small, rolled up receiving blanket or towel on either side of your baby's body and head, with the rolls outside of any straps, as seen below.

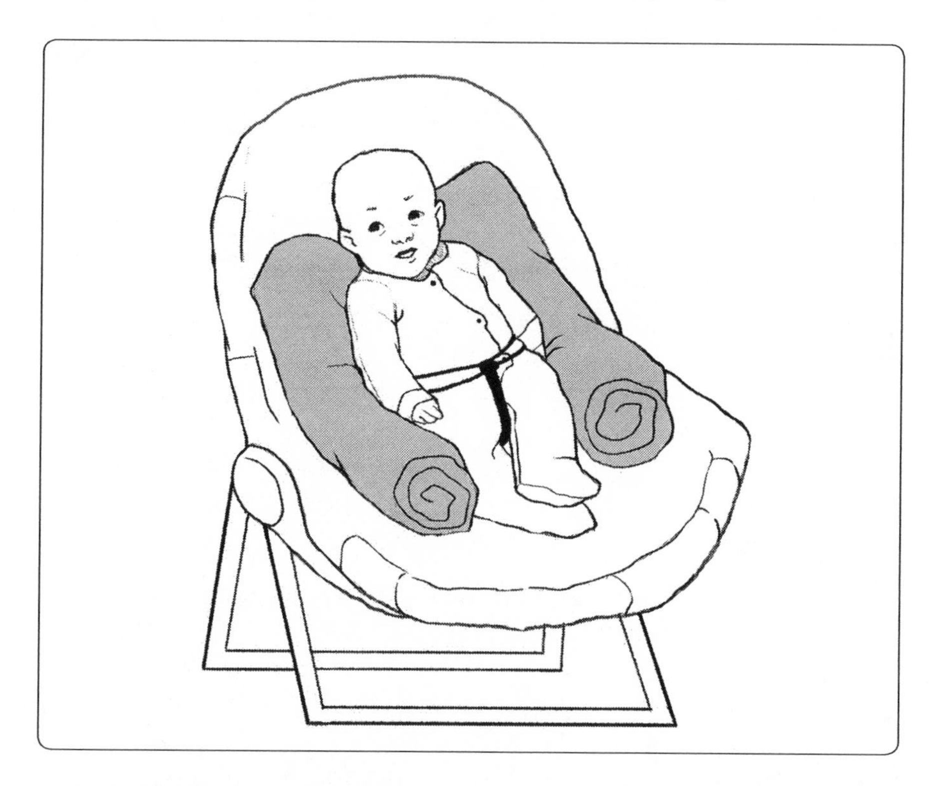

Optimal position for babies with reflux.

Rolls can be used to keep babies straight and centered in car seats, as well. However, car seat safety straps must remain snug against your baby's body. Apply rolls outside any straps after buckling your baby in the car seat. Always follow the instructions that came with the safety seat.

Place your baby flat on their back for sleep. Do not place your baby on their side or stomach for sleep as these positions increase the risk of sudden infant death syndrome (SIDS). Your baby's bed should be flat unless your doctor suggests another position.

Change your baby's diaper before or halfway through feeds. This is when the stomach is less full.

Use an inclined surface for diaper changes. Try a wedge or a pillow. When changing the diaper, roll your baby side to side, rather than lifting the legs.

Keep diapers loose. A tight-fitting diaper, straining on a bowel movement, or sitting in a hunched position can put extra pressure on your baby's stomach and increase reflux.

If the above first-line strategies do not improve your baby's symptoms after one to two weeks, talk to your baby's doctor. The "second-line" strategies that your doctor may suggest include formula change, adjustment to caloric density of the formula or breast milk, alternative sleep positions, elevating the head of the crib, and/or treatment with probiotics or medication.

Formula change. Your doctor may suggest a different formula or special dietary restrictions, such as dairy free, for breastfeeding mothers.

Caloric density change. Your doctor may adjust the concentration of what your baby is drinking, thereby changing caloric density. Drinking less volume of higher calories may reduce stomach stretching and reflux. On the other hand, higher-calorie feeds might slow down digestion, causing more reflux. Your doctor, nurse, or dietitian will guide you on making changes safely. Every baby responds differently. Monitor your baby's response and communicate with your health care team.

Alternate sleep position, elevating the head of the crib. Due to the risk of SIDS, these changes must be initiated by your doctor. Ask for specific instructions about alternate sleep positions. If your doctor suggests elevation of the head of the crib, ask how to do this safely. Bassinets are not safe to raise, as the mattress is too soft and the bassinet will be too unstable when tipped. A common way to raise the head of your baby's crib is to insert a wedge or folded blanket under the firm mattress, leaving the crib legs stable on the floor.

Probiotics. Probiotics help to improve gastrointestinal function and respiratory and allergy response, and to counter the negative effects of antibiotic use. Furthermore, these beneficial bacteria help the body to produce vitamins, absorb nutrients, and control overgrowth of bad bacteria and fungi. Probiotics have been tested in term and preterm babies, and children.

Reflux medications. Babies with GERD may benefit from medications to ease their pain. Medications are used to buffer gastric acid, reduce gastric acid secretion, and alter gastrointestinal movement or motility. Ask your doctor or pharmacist how to administer the medication for the best effect. Some medications work best when given on an empty stomach, such as thirty minutes before a feed. Once you start the medication, it may take two to ten days before you see any benefit. These medications may need to be increased as your baby's weight increases to maintain the effect. While these medications may lessen the pain associated with GERD, they may not stop the vomiting or other signs of reflux completely. But you should notice your baby is more comfortable, feeds better, and sleeps more soundly.

Keep in contact with your baby's doctor to regularly review reflux symptoms and management to determine the impact of medications on your baby's intake, growth, feeding, and sleep.

Impact of reflux on parents. Many times we have witnessed the challenges parents face when their baby has reflux. Reflux may affect the parent-infant relationship. The workload from increased laundry and cleaning vomit from chairs, car seats, cribs, rugs, and so on is certainly inconvenient. Parents feel stressed during feeds, not knowing if their baby will feel comfortable, will vomit, or be screaming in pain afterward.

Parents become scared when their baby is not feeding well and is throwing up and may go to any extent to get their baby to feed. Sometimes parents focus too much on feeding volumes and weight gain and resort to forced feeding. The feeding experience then becomes stressful and unpleasant for baby and parents and can affect the parents' ability to bond and attach with their baby.

♥ *I remember putting my baby on my shoulder to burp him and hearing a huge splash on the floor behind me. Then I would be in panic mode because I wouldn't know how much volume he had lost, if he would take a top-up or if I should move his next feed up to compensate. He would also have spells where he would have a small but acidic spit-up and then his body would go completely stiff and he would arch his back. During those spells, we could tell he was in intense pain.*

I fight with my baby until he is worn out. I hold his arms down and swaddle him tightly or he will push the bottle away. I hate doing this but feeding and weight gain are so important. Finally, he gets sleepy and then he will feed. The entire feed takes 1½ hours. It is exhausting.

If you and your baby are experiencing stressful feedings like the two described above, begin first-line reflux strategies immediately. If there is no improvement or if you notice symptoms of severe reflux, discuss this with your family doctor right away. The doctor may want to start treatment or reevaluate the medication if your baby is already being treated for reflux. You may even be referred to a feeding specialist who will help work on any problematic behaviors.

We did not take the decision to put our son on medication lightly. We were aware of the fact that he was already on caffeine, iron, vitamin supplements, and fortifiers for his milk and we really were uncomfortable with the idea of introducing another medication into his body. In the end, we did our research and discussed at length with our nurse and pediatrician and decided that the benefits of taking the meds were significant and in our son's best interest. He took Omeprazole for about six months and now handles all liquids and solids very well. Every case of reflux is different and every family has a different schedule, so I recommend talking to your care team about what is best for your baby.

ACTION PLAN: Reflux

Try these strategies for living with a baby with reflux:

- Keep a reflux log or diary. Your observations are very important in recognizing and treating reflux. Keep a written record of what you do from feeding to feeding and your baby's response. Note what works and what doesn't. Recording every symptom of reflux and how much volume is lost over a period of time can bring to light the seriousness of the reflux. Details from this diary will help your doctor make decisions about treatment and other aspects of your baby's care.
- Learn all you can. Learn about reflux and possible treatment options. There are many things to try before adding medication. The more you know, the better the reflux can be managed. Your baby will give you the signs if things are working or not.
- Do a CPR training course. Babies with reflux sometimes have choking episodes at home. The CPR course will prepare you to manage an emergency situation while 911 is on the way.
- Get a second opinion. There are many different approaches to treating reflux. Don't be afraid to advocate for your baby and ask for a second opinion.
- Take a break. Managing reflux can be exhausting. Severe reflux can impact family quality of life. You really need support and the ability to take a break. Self-care improves your mental state, and also helps you refuel and be the best parent you can be.

Milk-free diet and cow's milk protein allergy

Cow's milk protein allergy (CMPA) occurs when your baby's immune system reacts to the protein found in cow's milk. Cow's milk proteins are found in breast milk, formula, and some fortifiers. This reaction can cause injury in the stomach and intestines and symptoms similar to reflux. Babies may also have blood or mucus in their stools.

CMPA is suspected in babies who have family members with cow's milk protein allergy or symptoms such as diarrhea, blood in the stool, red and itchy patches of skin (atopic dermatitis), and runny nose. As well, up to 25 percent of babies with reflux have CMPA.

For formula-supplemented babies with suspected CMPA, the doctor may recommend a time-limited trial of a hypoallergenic infant formula. Improvement should be seen within a couple weeks after trying a cow's-milk-free diet. For babies receiving breast milk, the doctor may suggest the mother adopt a dairy-free diet and pump for a limited time before resuming breastfeeding. Label your stored breast milk with "contains milk" for later use. Breastfeeding mothers should talk to their doctor or dietitian for details on dairy-free diets and vitamin D or calcium supplementation.

CMPA may not last forever. Most infants will outgrow it by one year of age. The method to reintroduce cow's milk proteins is unknown. A trial of reintroduction may be initiated around six months of age. Talk to your doctor about how and when to try reintroducing cow's milk protein.

Final Thoughts

Tummy troubles are common, especially in the first year home. The preemie's digestive system is immature. This can result in burping, tooting, spitting up, and pooping issues. Many simple strategies to reduce signs and symptoms can be tried at home, but they may not solve the problems completely. Sometimes it just takes time. As the gastrointestinal system matures, the troubles tend to go away.

♥ *My baby developed reflux once home, with medium- to large-sized vomits after every feeding. We ruled out gassiness and constipation as a cause. Her feeding skills were good, so it wasn't that. We tried everything—smaller, more frequent feeds, pacing, burp breaks, and holding her upright after feeds—nothing worked. Then she started to be irritable and seemed uncomfortable after feeds, with dry swallows, squirming, and arching, and I was finding feedings stressful and challenging.*

♥ *She started on medication for reflux, but after two weeks nothing improved. She became very fussy at the sight of the bottle or when we tried to put her in the feeding position. She would turn her head away and put her hands in front of her face.*

The next step was to try a two- to four-week trial of a new hypoallergenic formula and a cow's milk protein–free diet for me. Within two weeks her regurgitations reduced to occasional wet burps and no major spit-ups. We were overjoyed!

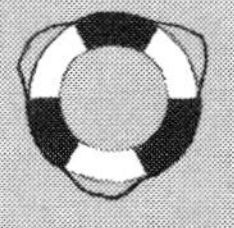

EXPERT TIPS

Here are the key strategies to navigate the journey

- Expect some tummy troubles over the first year, as these are very common.
- Use simple strategies to relieve your baby's gas.
- Learn the difference between infrequent passing of stool and constipation.
- Use our simple strategies to ease infrequent stooling.
- Watch for signs of dehydration with vomiting or diarrhea.
- Know the difference between spit-ups and reflux.
- Rule out other factors that can contribute to reflux.
- Several lifestyle and feeding changes can help control or resolve reflux.
- Try the conservative, first-line strategies for reflux before considering medication.
- Discuss second-line reflux strategies with your doctor if reflux persists.
- Communicate regularly with your health care team about reflux progress.

6

CHARTING YOUR BABY'S COURSE
Behavior and Development

NOW THAT you and baby are home, you can really "get to know" your baby's temperament, behavior, and communication style. Communication and behavior can be different for premature babies than it is for full-term babies, due to preemies' immaturity. The more you understand your baby's behavior, the easier it is to respond appropriately to their needs. Preemie development is also a common source of worry for parents as babies born preterm run the risk for developmental delay. You play an extremely important role in your baby's development. Cultivating a loving relationship and providing an environment rich in learning opportunities can help your baby reach their potential.

This chapter begins with an introduction to temperament and communication. Consider this a language lesson. We also address strategies for parents to calm fussy, crying babies. And we present an in-depth review of development from "term" to one year corrected age. You will learn the importance of monitoring and applying corrected age to your baby's development. Our detailed development and play suggestions will help you stimulate your baby's development and, more importantly, enjoy this wonderful time with your baby.

♥ *We had heard preemies were more difficult, more challenging to care for and parent. That was our boy. Having already had a full-term baby, we knew he was different. He cried louder and longer. He was hard to calm down. If I missed his early feeding cues, he'd turn into a monster. It would take ten minutes to calm him down so that he could feed without choking. Changing his diaper made him crazy. He was really irritable, especially on days when we had appointments or errands to run. He hated the swing. He never slept long. We tried all kinds of things, but the only thing that worked was holding him. The front baby pack was a lifesaver. I could strap him to me and move around.*

It took us until he was six months corrected age to figure him out. He was a really sensitive boy. New things and change were hard for him. He was such a different baby when we stayed home. Once we figured out what he liked and disliked, we were able to finally find peace. He loved it when I dimmed the lights and we listened to soft music. Nothing better than a quiet, content baby.

Behavior

A baby's behavior or way that they interact with others and the world depends on many factors, including their natural temperament, ability to communicate, and reaction to what is happening around them. Premature babies are challenged by their immature nervous system and body and may present with confusing behaviors.

Temperament

Temperament describes a baby's personal "style," their way of being, how they approach and react to the world. Temperament influences a baby's behavior and the way they interact with others. Understanding temperament helps you identify your baby's strengths and the supports they need to succeed in their relationships and the environment as they mature and grow.

You may hear the terms *temperament* and *personality* used interchangeably. These terms do have similar meanings. Temperament is innate, inborn, or develops naturally. We can control our temperament, but we cannot learn it. Personality is built upon our temperament, and developed through years of education, experiences, and social activities. Personality includes our behaviors, feelings, and thoughts. Adults can control or modify our personality through choices, education, or experiences. Since babies have very little education or life experience, we will use "temperament" and "personality" synonymously in this book.

Some babies are easy or flexible and tend to be happy, regular in sleeping and eating, adaptable, calm, and not easily upset. Others are active or feisty and may be fussy, irregular in sleeping and eating, easily distracted or upset by noise and stimulation, and reactive. Other babies are slow to warm up or cautious and may be less active, fussy, withdrawn, or negatively reactive in new situations. And some babies have a combination of all of these temperaments, depending on the time of day, how much sleep they've had, and their mood. Not too different from any of us.

♥ *My baby was irritable all the time, He would fuss and cry all day, especially when we changed his diaper or did tummy time. He was my hard baby. And my other baby was so easy, calm, and quiet.*

♥ *All along my girl has been quiet and shy. That's just who she is. I learned how to help her warm up in new situations. I give her time and encourage her, and I have learned that she needs support when doing something new. Transitions are hard for her. She is very loving and cuddly. I wouldn't change her for anything.*

You will get to know your baby's temperament over time. Temperament evolves gradually. You will learn triggers for your baby's reactions and strategies that work for your baby. When you notice that your baby has become unusually quiet or very fussy, be sure there is no health reason for this change.

Communication

All babies, even preemies, communicate through their behavior. The more you understand your baby's behavior, the easier it is to respond appropriately, which may improve their physical, social, and emotional growth. Your baby will not have to waste energy communicating their needs because you understand their signals.

Babies use two kinds of behavior to communicate: approach and withdrawal signals.

Approach signals. These are behaviors babies use when ready to interact with you. Cooing, smiling, or making eye contact are positive signs. Approach signals indicate that your baby likes whatever is happening in the moment and they want it to continue. They are a GO sign.

Withdrawal signals. These are behaviors that babies use when they need a break. These include crying, fussing, or back-arching. Perhaps they are tired and need a rest from interacting with you, need the feed to stop, or are uncomfortable and need some help. Withdrawal signals indicate that your baby does not like what is happening in the moment and wants it to stop. They are a STOP sign.

Babies often start communicating with subtle cues and then move to stronger signals if their needs are not met. For example, a hungry baby might start to fuss and smack their lips. If you do not respond, they may advance to crying and more activity.

Younger premature babies tend to have subtler cues at first, and parents may easily miss them. Older babies exhibit stronger signals. Your baby will learn to trust you when their needs are met before they fall back to sleep or before they become too upset.

Approach and withdrawal signals

Approach Signals	Withdrawal Signals
Subtle • Eyes wide and bright • Eyebrow-raising • Finger-folding • Fist to mouth • Head-raising • Hands open and relaxed • Feeding posture • Body movement	Subtle • Frowning and wrinkled forehead • Looking away • Hiccups • Grimace • Tense straight fingers • Eyes squeezed shut • Yawning • Lip compression • Sneezing
Strong • Eye-to-eye contact • Looking at your face • Turning head toward you • Sucking • Reaching to you • Feeding sounds • Smiling • Talking, cooing, babbling • Smooth, regular body movements	Strong • Back-arching • Spitting up • Crying • Fussing • Halt hand • Falling asleep • Pulling away • Coughing • Choking or gagging

Your baby's pattern of signals may change from day to day. Looking at you can be a difficult cue to read. Is your baby learning about you, curious about you, or hungry? A few signals grouped together gives a stronger message. Eye contact, turning toward you, and sucking are pretty strong signals that your baby is hungry. Back arching, spitting up, and pulling away are strong signals that your baby has had enough food or stimulation. In time, you will become comfortable interpreting your baby's communication.

Fussiness

Every baby is unique but preemie babies are known to be fussier and more difficult to settle.

Premature babies have been described as:

- less adaptive to new people and surroundings;
- less regular in their feeding and sleeping patterns;
- more likely to cry;
- more difficult to soothe;
- more withdrawn.

Prematurity impacts behavior. A difficult temperament is more common among preemies who are smaller and younger at birth. They often leave the hospital at or close to their due date and have unpredictable waking and sleeping times, irregular feeding patterns, limited or disorganized responses, less adaptability, and low energy levels. Usually, they just need some time to catch up.

Environment plays a role, too. When overstimulated, some preemies become easily agitated, and some become the opposite. They disengage to block out stimulation. During their first few months and years of life, a preemie is more easily overstimulated than a term baby. Be aware of things in your home environment that might overstimulate your baby, such as loud noises, other children playing or running around, too much handling. This is especially important during feeding. According to parents, for the majority of preemies, their temperament stabilizes by the time they are ready for preschool.

The relationship between you and your baby is very important. This is sometimes referred to as "goodness of fit," which describes how well a baby's temperament meshes with the key people in their life and how likable these people consider the baby to be. Some parents adjust quickly to the needs of a demanding premature baby and feel satisfaction from parenting. Some parents struggle to like the behaviors they see, and they think their baby is too demanding or too fussy. While it is normal not to love everything your baby does, it is not normal for you to be upset, angry, or overwhelmed by your baby's behavior. Your experiences with your baby should be primarily positive. If you are struggling with your baby's behavior or temperament, reach out for help from friends and family and community resources (support groups, church, health care providers/programs). Fussy babies are very time-consuming. Take care of yourself, too.

A common pattern among all babies is to be fussy during the evening for one to three hours. You may notice that your baby wants to be held and fed frequently.

> ♥ *We call it the "witching hour." Everyone is going crazy. My older kids are cranky. Baby is cranky. I'm cranky. We buckle down and ensure everyone is fed, clean, and ready for a good night's sleep.*

Awareness of your baby's likes and dislikes will help build positive interactions between you and your baby and the surroundings. The better you know your baby, the better these interactions will be. A positive relationship between you and your baby is important, as it can have lasting effects on your baby's development and health.

See the section below for the action plan to help calm a fussy baby.

Crying

At the time of discharge, most parents of premature babies would say that their baby is quiet and does not cry very much. For preemies, crying starts closer to term, or your due date. At that time, your baby is more mature and therefore capable of communicating through action and crying. Don't misinterpret crying as their opinion of life at home.

> ♥ *My girl was so quiet in the NICU. All the nurses commented on how lovely she was. But at home, she cried more. I thought she didn't like being at home, and I was so relieved to hear that crying starts at term. Once I knew that crying is a form of communication, I could do something to respond.*

For full-term newborns, crying reaches a peak around two months of age and then eases. The peak of crying for premature babies tends to occur later, at three to four months corrected age, and then settles. This can be a confusing time for parents as they learn what the crying means.

Crying is a strong form of communication, one of the STOP signals that indicate your baby needs help. But what do they need? Crying could signal hunger, discomfort, a wet diaper, pain, overstimulation, loneliness, or feeling overtired.

You will learn to interpret your baby's cry and come to know the reasons your baby usually cries. As your baby matures, the cry will vary according to the reasons for the cry. Around two to three months corrected age, the characteristics of your baby's cry will begin to associate with specific needs and the urgency of these. As such, you will learn to differentiate a hunger cry from an overtired cry, a dirty-diaper cry from a distressed cry, an "I'm fussy" cry from an "I need you right now" cry. You will be mastering your baby's language.

Particularly with premature babies, sometimes there may be no identifiable reason for crying. Often your baby's cues are unclear, and you are not sure whether to play or cuddle, feed or sleep, soothe, or leave them alone. This happens to all parents and can be very frustrating. Try our suggestions for soothing.

ACTION PLAN: Fussy or Crying Baby

Try these strategies to calm a fussy or crying baby:

- Calm your baby with your touch by cuddling or swaddle snugly in a blanket (see chapter 3).
- Gently rub or pat your baby's back.
- Hold your baby close to your body.
- Offer skin-to-skin cuddles.
- Carry your baby in a front pack while you perform daily activities.
- Give baby a massage, including tummy massage to relieve gas and abdominal pain.
- Feed your baby if they seem hungry.
- Offer a soother.

- Speak or sing to baby with a calm, gentle voice. Babies learn the sound of their parents' voices.
- Turn on a white noise machine, radio, vacuum cleaner, clothes dryer, dishwasher, or overhead fan.
- Provide gentle, rhythmical movement, such carefully jiggling or rocking baby, going for a drive or a walk in the stroller, sitting in a bouncy chair or swing.
- Place rolled-up blankets beside your baby when in a bouncy chair or swing to aid feelings of security.
- Spend time in a quiet, dark room with your baby. Dim the lights, turn off the TV or radio, or turn down the volume. Some babies are overstimulated by too much light or sound.
- Avoid overstimulation of your baby by you, your family, or friends.
- Ensure that your baby is not crying because of a medical problem. If your baby continues to cry, seek advice from a doctor.

A crying baby can be stressful for many parents. It is very challenging to care for a baby who fusses and cries a lot. If you are concerned about your baby's crying and these suggestions are not helping to settle your baby, talk to your doctor, nurse, or health care provider.

ACTION PLAN: Care for Parents

Try these strategies for *you* as you care for a fussy or crying baby:

- If you ever feel angry, frustrated, or out of control, put your baby down in their crib and take a five- to ten-minute break.
- Use relaxation techniques to calm yourself (for example, breathe deeply and slowly).
- Ask a friend, relative, or neighbor to care for your baby while you take a break.

- Regularly take some time off to prevent burnout. Don't feel guilty about this, as it is for your baby's good, as well. You cannot pour from an empty vessel! By relaxing and replenishing your emotional energy, you will be better able to cope with your baby. (See chapter 7 for more self-care ideas.)
- If you have a fussy baby or one who cries a lot, choose your babysitters carefully. Find people who have lots of experience with small, fussy, or crying babies. If you're not sure that someone has the patience and maturity to care for a crying baby, don't leave your child alone with them.
- Develop a safety plan for times when you are overwhelmed by your crying baby, for example, grandma, close friend, or a neighbor. Know who you can call for support. Ask your community health nurse for suggestions for other resources.
- Never shake your baby and tell everyone who cares for your baby to never, ever shake a baby.

Developmental Considerations

For many babies, development seems to happen naturally. They learn to sit, roll, crawl, talk, and walk. Every baby's development sequence and pace is unique. Parents should not fret if their baby does not reach every milestone at the time listed on a developmental checklist. Sometimes a baby will be slower in one area of development while they excel in another. Keep this in mind when you refer to the checklists later in this chapter. They are only a guide.

There is so much a parent can do to foster development. A baby's head control will strengthen with parent help. A baby will be more interested in crawling or walking with parent encouragement. You have the power to make a big difference in your baby's developmental progress. This is particularly important for babies who may be at risk of developmental delay, such as babies born prematurely or babies with large intraventricular hemorrhage (bleeding into the brain). Stimulating exercises are suggested below. Track your baby's developmental progress, starting with zero to two months corrected age. As your baby ages, move to the next section for information about what to look for and what you can do to stimulate development.

Chronologic age versus corrected age. You must begin an exploration of infant development with an understanding of your baby's "true" age, called their "corrected age" or "adjusted age." Refer to chapter 1 for a detailed explanation of chronologic age and corrected age. In short, chronologic age refers to the actual date your baby was born. Corrected age refers to your baby's age according to your due date. A baby born three months early, five months ago, is two months corrected age.

Do not make the mistake of applying full-term developmental stages to your premature baby. For example, if a baby born three months early is not standing or walking one year later, a parent might be concerned. But since this baby was born three months early, we know this baby is not truly one year old. This baby is nine months corrected age and is, therefore, appropriately working on crawling. This baby should not be expected to fulfill the developmental tasks of a one-year-old child. Misinterpreting your baby's corrected age will cause you undue stress and worry. Be informed about corrected age so that you can correctly monitor your baby and use appropriate play activities. By using your baby's "true" or corrected age, you are essentially giving your baby credit for their degree of prematurity. We cannot speed up development. Development happens when each body system is ready.

If your baby is quite premature, health care professionals will use your baby's corrected age when evaluating growth and development. Using the corrected age is important when monitoring the development of babies born more than one month early.

If your premature baby was born less than one month early, your baby's developmental progress will likely not be greatly impacted. If your baby was born at thirty-six to thirty-nine weeks' gestation, feel free to jump straight to the section on developmental milestone details.

Parents of babies more than one month premature often ask how to respond when someone asks how old the baby is. Your response is up to you, but consider these three responses as demonstrated by a chronologically six-month-old baby, who is actually four months corrected age:

1. "She's six months old." (Give your baby's chronologic age and watch the questioner's puzzled face when they try to understand why your baby doesn't look or act like a six-month-old.)
2. "She's six months old, but she was born two months early. That's why she looks like a four-month-old." (This is nice and succinct. It might raise a few questions, but this short statement avoids the puzzled look!)
3. "She's four months old." (Your baby's corrected age is their true age. To another family member or stranger, the corrected age will make sense.)

You can stop correcting your baby's age whenever it feels most comfortable to you. Once your baby is able to walk around your house and go up and down stairs, you won't be thinking of their corrected age anymore.

Many health care professionals stop using corrected age around three years of age, as that is when most body systems have caught up to their chronologic age. Some health care professionals will continue to use corrected age for up to five years for babies born less than twenty-eight weeks' gestation.

Developmental delay

While more and more premature babies are living without severe or moderate disabilities, the risk of developmental delay in premature babies still remains, and is greater in very premature babies. The longer your baby has gestated before birth, the lesser the risk of developmental challenge. If your baby was born at twenty-eight weeks or earlier, health care professionals recommend close monitoring of developmental progress until your baby is three to five years old.

The good news is that most premature babies reach the same developmental milestones as their full-term peers in two to three years. After that, any differences in size or development may be due to individual differences or environment, rather than premature birth. Some very small babies take longer to catch up.

Early identification and intervention are key to minimizing or preventing developmental delay. You know your baby best and often you will be the one to pick up when your baby is not progressing. The sooner a delay is identified, the sooner treatment can start. Delays in treatment may cause your baby to become behind developmentally.

Top two strategies to promote early development

There are two key interventions that parents can do during the first few months at home that will have the biggest impact on encouraging their baby's early social and physical development.

1. **You!** Parents are the first and most important intervention. Parental presence is a powerful promoter of infant bonding, trust, security, social attachment, behavior, and mental development. Your baby needs your touch and voice more than any other toy. You communicate back and forth with your baby. These are known as "serve and return" interactions and are critical for brain

growth and development. Give your baby a signal (smile or stick out your tongue), and baby learns to respond the same way. Then, when baby gives you a signal, you respond. Responding with a positive action teaches your baby to continue engaging with you. Responding with a negative action or no response conveys a negative message and discourages the interaction. There is nothing complicated about this strategy. Keep it simple. Do what comes naturally.

ACTION PLAN: Early Development

Try these strategies to promote attachment and baby development:

- Gently stroke your baby's skin.
- Gaze into your baby's eyes.
- Smile at your baby.
- Sing songs, recite nursery rhymes.
- Read a book or talk out loud.
- Give skin-to-skin cuddles.
- Tickle and massage your baby.
- Talk to your baby while you are caring for them and when they start "talking" (babbling or cooing).
- Modify the intonations of your voice as you talk or read. In other words, make your conversation "interesting" to hear.
- Spend time just "being with" your baby.
- Have fun playtime every day.

Be in the moment with your baby and try not to think of the other things you need to do. Spending time with your baby should be quality time and is an investment in your baby's mental well-being.

2. **Tummy time.** This is the second-most important development activity for newly discharged babies. You will see tummy time recommended as a strategy at each stage of our development checklist until baby starts to crawl.

Tummy time will help strengthen your baby's neck, shoulder, and arms. This is important because development starts at the top of the body and proceeds downward. Without strong head control and upper body strength, your baby's development will not proceed well. Tummy time is the best way to encourage physical development in the first several months beyond term.

It can be hard to find a good time for tummy time. Try it during the few minutes before a feeding when your baby's tummy is empty. Tummy time after feeds might not be a good idea as it may cause your baby to vomit. After bath time, while you dry your baby's back, maybe work on tummy time. If your baby is awake while you are watching television, both of you can get on the floor for a few exercises during commercials.

♥ *I was overwhelmed with feeding and pumping and trying to get some rest. I never seemed to find time to do tummy time, or I completely forgot. Then my nurse suggested tummy time after diaper changes. While I was throwing out the diaper and washing my hands, he got a few minutes of tummy time in his crib. Then he got at least five practices a day.*

Build multiple tummy times into your daily routines. Start with very short practice sessions and gradually increase the duration. Work up to ten to fifteen minutes of tummy time at least three times a day. Eventually, this will be enjoyable and part of play time.

ACTION PLAN: Tummy Time

Engage your baby in tummy time every day. Here's how to do it:

- Do tummy time on the floor or crib or on your chest. A bed or couch are too soft for this exercise.
- Place your baby on their stomach on a blanket.
- With your baby's face looking down toward the blanket, talk to your baby in one ear to encourage your baby to turn toward your voice and face. When your baby turns to face you, praise them and smile. Repeat the exercise on the other side.

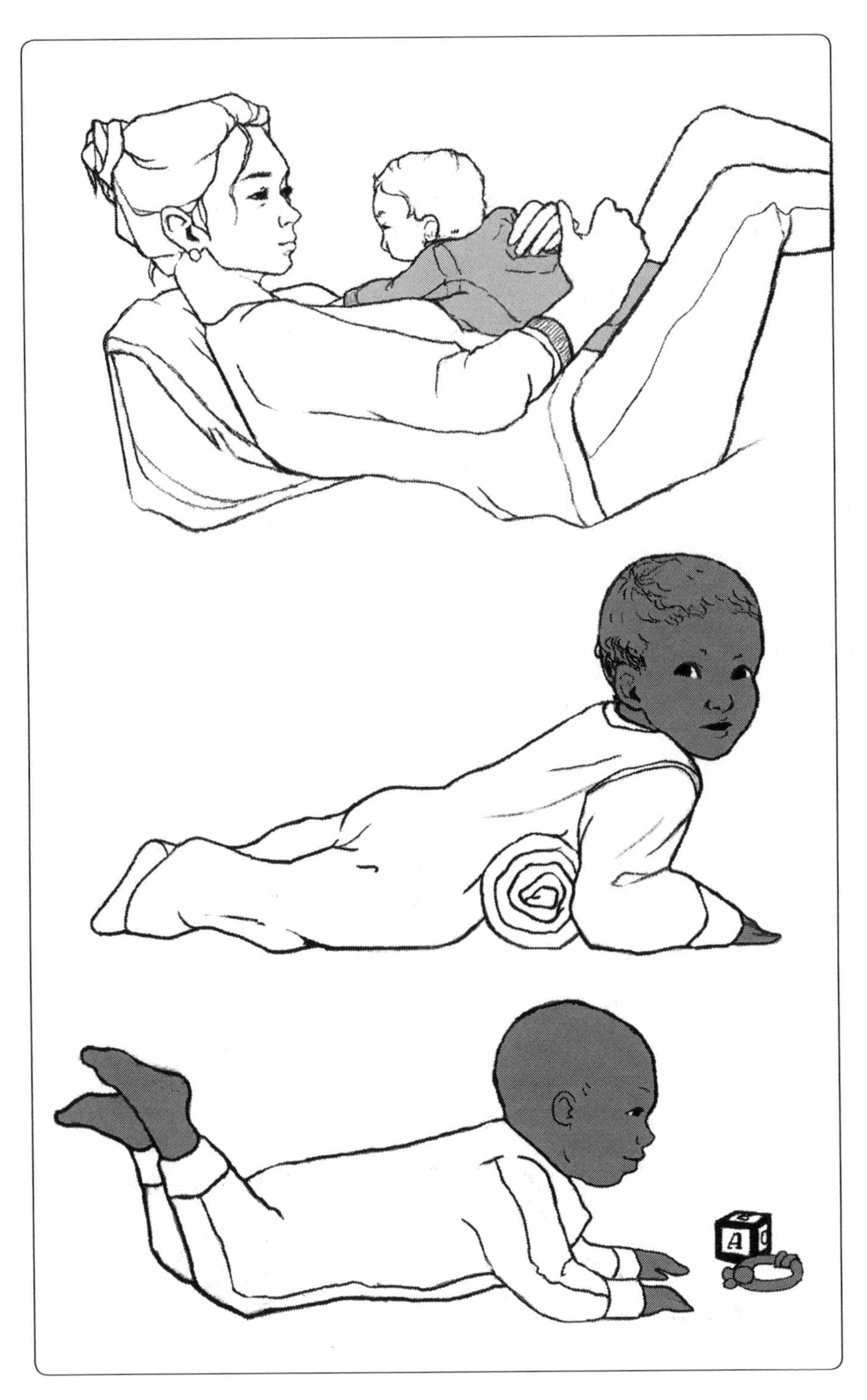

Three different tummy time techniques to support your baby's development.

- If your baby cries during tummy time or if it is challenging, put a large roll under the armpits to support your baby's chest as shown in the illustration above. Use a wedge or breastfeeding pillow for supervised tummy time. Try it over your leg.
- Lay your baby on your chest while you slowly recline until you are flat on the floor with your baby doing tummy time on your chest as shown in the illustration above. Don't wear clothing with buttons or zippers that could hurt your baby.
- Get down on the floor with your baby. Looking at your face might be the encouragement they need.
- Use a rattle or toy to encourage your baby to lift and turn their head. This is particularly effective for babies beyond two months corrected age.
- Get excited! Motivate them to lift their head.

Tummy time is the most important playtime exercise you can do to encourage physical development in the early months. You'll be doing tummy time with your baby for more than six months. Make it fun!

Play groups and enrichment programs

Play groups and enrichment programs are not necessary but can be a fun way to spend time with your baby. Some parents report that they "normalize" your baby.

♥ *It's time to get out with the rest of the world. Enough prematurity. She might as well start hanging out with the kids that she will go to kindergarten with. She may be small, but they will soon learn that she's as smart and chatty as any of them. And maybe seeing the other kids run and tumble about will motivate her to be more active.*

You may find programs on development, play, music, swimming, baby massage, baby gym, or socialization, and programs designed for babies born prematurely. Remember to register for programs according to baby's corrected age.

Developmental Guide

The remainder of this chapter is dedicated to corrected age developmental milestones, parent stimulation suggestions, and warning signs for these time frames:

- Zero to two months
- Two to four months
- Four to six months
- Six to nine months
- Nine to twelve months

The range of normal development is wide. Infants and children reach milestones in unique ways, along individual time frames. If you are concerned about your baby's development, speak to your baby's doctor.

If your baby shows a developmental delay in physical, vocal, or social areas, speak to your baby's doctor about early intervention physiotherapy and occupational therapy/speech-language therapy. Babies who are at high risk of developmental delay, for example, those who were very sick in the NICU or born less than twenty-eight weeks' gestation, will benefit from physiotherapy and occupational therapy. No need to wait for developmental problems. Research has shown that early intervention improves baby outcomes.

Parents of premature babies sometimes get too caught up in vigilant monitoring. You've seen your babies at their most fragile and sick and your parental instincts to nurture and protect fired up. Tracking development can become a source of work and worry. But development is supposed to be fun for you and your baby. You want to feel joy when you see your baby reach, roll, or walk. Your baby would want you to enjoy their accomplishments. With that in mind, we've written the developmental milestones in your baby's voice. Let your baby tell you how amazing they are!

Zero to two months old corrected age

I have now reached and passed my original due date. Even though it's been weeks or months since my birth, I am just a newborn, developmentally. In these two months, I will learn much about my body and you. I am excited to spend lots of time with you. Thank you for keeping me safe.

Let's look at the developmental skills I will learn from zero to two months and the strategies you can use to support me.

Movement (Zero to two months)

- ☑ I am a wiggler! I like to move my arms and legs. My movements might be jerky at first and will become smoother.
- ☑ My limbs move symmetrically. This means that my right and left arms and right and left legs move in similar ways.
- ☑ My legs move in and out together. At the end of this developmental stage, you notice that my legs start to move one at a time.
- ☑ When I lie quietly, you notice that my legs and arms are usually bent, like a frog's limbs.
- ☑ When I sit on your lap, my back is rounded.
- ☑ My hands are closed in a fist at first because I have a hand grasp reflex. Gradually this reflex relaxes and my hands open.
- ☑ Usually, I move my fingers all at once, as I don't know how to move each finger individually yet.
- ☑ I make funny facial expressions while I sleep. You might see me smile or look angry, sad, or surprised.
- ☑ I startle at loud noises. I extend my arms and/or legs all at once and then pull them toward my body. I might cry.
- ☑ At the end of this stage, I start to smile at you. Smile back at me please!
- ☑ At the end of this stage, I start bringing my hands to my chest and face. I can scratch my face so keep my nails short.

Movement Action Plan (Zero to two months)

- Handle your baby gently.
- Hold your baby to convey love and security.
- Place your baby in a swing or bouncy chair, but don't leave them there for a long time, as they will develop a flat spot at the back of their head.
- Swaddle your baby's legs and arms if the activity of their limbs keeps them awake. If your baby likes their arms out, swaddle their body and legs.
- Give gentle massages.

Behavior (Zero to two months)

☑ I sleep a lot. My sleep is a bit restless and noisy. I move my legs and arms frequently and open and close my eyes. I make little fussy noises that are very different from my crying sounds. Sometimes you think I'm waking up and then I go back to sleep.

☑ I can only handle brief periods of social interaction when I'm awake. It's easy for me to be overstimulated.

☑ I calm down when you meet my needs, for example, feed me, change my diaper, or comfort me.

☑ Bath time might not be my favorite yet. I might get upset when I feel wet and cold.

☑ At the end of stage, I'm more alert and I stay awake for longer periods.

Behavior Action Plan (Zero to two months)

- Touch your baby. Stroke the head, chest, tummy, legs, and arms. Touch is calming, helps your baby learn about their body, and promotes parent-baby bonding. Use a variety of touch sensations, such as different textures, bumpy toys, smooth objects, and different temperatures.
- Provide skin-to-skin contact to help your baby calm down.
- Carry your baby in a front pack to promote calming and bonding, and to free up your arms.
- Respond to your baby's cry, as this is their form of communication. At this stage, your response develops infant-parent trust. You don't need to pick up your baby every time they make a sound.
- Sometimes they just need to hear you, feel your touch, be re-swaddled, or have a diaper change.
- Watch for signs of overstimulation. Restlessness, crying, arching, or making an unhappy facial expression are signs to stop the activity.

Head Control (Zero to two months)

☑ I cannot hold my head steady. This is called "head lag" and is normal at this stage. My head flops forward or backward or tips to the side.

☑ My head control is very weak when I'm tired.

☑ When I am put into "tummy time" position with my face down, I can turn my head to the side.

☑ It is hard for me to lift my head during tummy time.

☑ When you put me in "airplane" position, I can hold my head for a short time and then it becomes too heavy for me.

☑ At the end of this stage, I start to self-correct my head control. My head might bob forward but I can bring it up most of the time.

Head Control Action Plan (Zero to two months)

- Support your baby's head.
- When your baby is being held or lying down, ensure their head is in alignment with their body and not tipped to the side or forward.
- Routinely change your baby's position in their crib every night or two so that they change the direction of their gaze. If your baby is in a bassinet, turn the bassinette around every night or two. (See "Head shape and plagiocephaly" in chapter 3.)
- Practice tummy time several times a day. (See tummy time suggestions above.)
- Once baby turns their head to each side well, work on "tummy time push-ups." Lay baby on their tummy on a blanket, placing their hands near their shoulders so that they can use them to push up. Direct baby's nose downward and talk to them near the top of their head to encourage them to look up. Baby will probably lift with head and neck only.
- Use "airplane" position to build baby's neck muscles (see illustration below). With baby facing toward the floor, cradle them in your arms, supporting their torso. Let baby hold their head, arms, and legs by themselves. This is hard for baby, so only do this for short periods, stopping when your baby's head drops.
- At the end of this stage, practice sitting to develop head control. When your baby is wide awake, position them on your thighs facing you. Your legs should be on a stool or coffee table so that you and baby are at eye level. Be encouraging with your eyes, smiles, and voice. Support the back and monitor whether baby can hold their head steady and midline. Your baby will get better at this with practice.

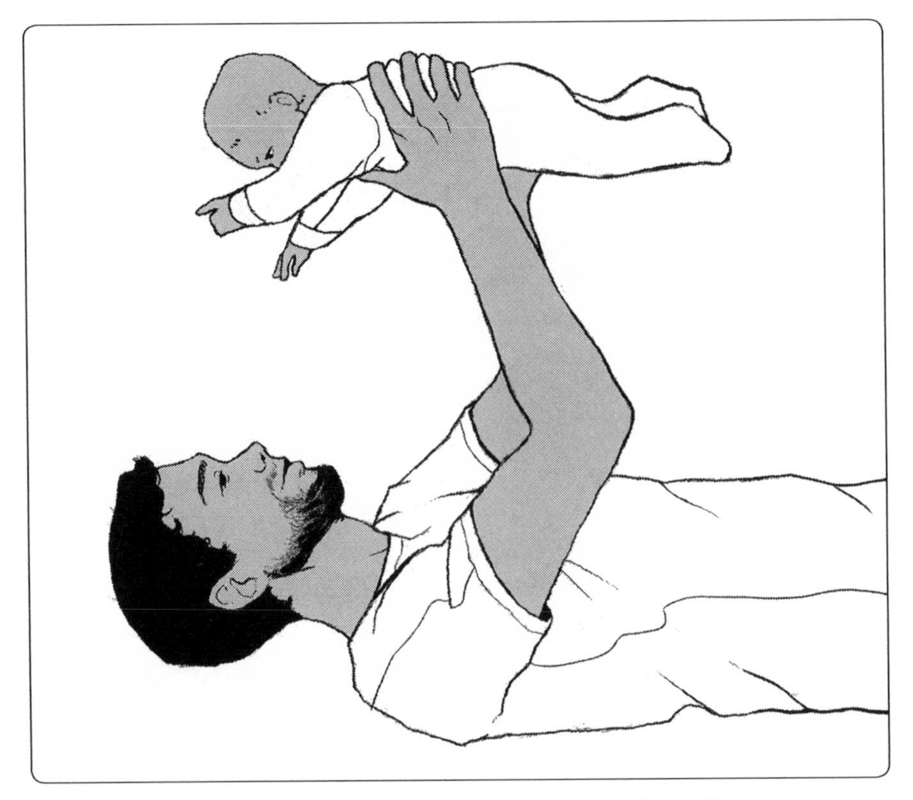

Airplane position: this is challenging for baby at this stage, but they will improve with practice.

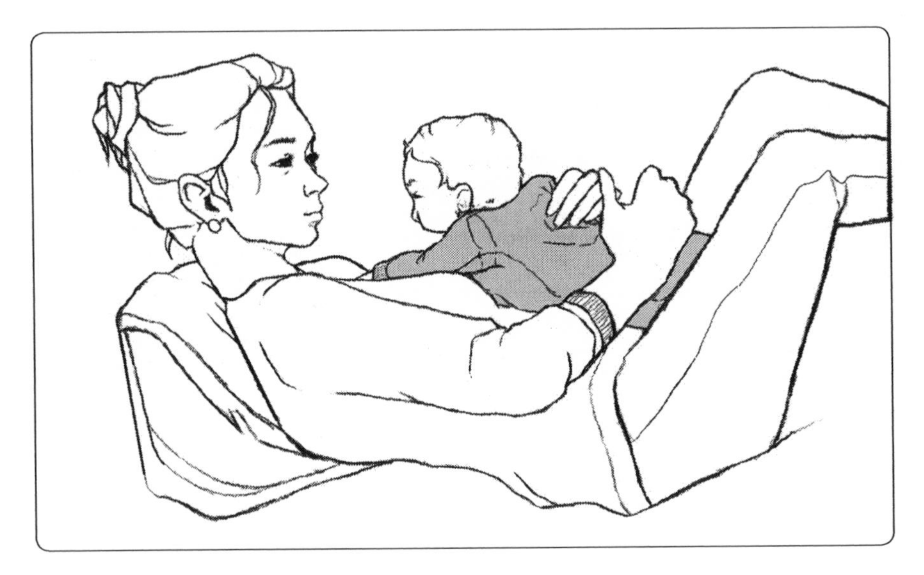

Your baby should be at eye level so they can look directly into your eyes.

Vision (Zero to two months)

- ☑ I can see you when you hold me twenty to fifty centimeters (eight to nineteen inches) from your face.
- ☑ I love to look at faces and probably prefer faces to toys at this age. I might look at toys for a very short time.
- ☑ I like to make eye contact.
- ☑ I like to look at highly contrasted patterns, for example, patterns that are light and dark.
- ☑ I watch faces or toys with my eyes. I might not turn my head to watch them yet.
- ☑ I am cross-eyed from time to time. I am learning how to use my many eye muscles.
- ☑ At the end of this stage, I start to watch moving objects and people and to see further. I might notice objects on the wall or people walking by.

Vision Action Plan (Zero to two months)

- Hold your baby about fifty centimeters (nineteen inches) from your face and let them look into your eyes and study every feature of your face and head.
- Smile at your baby. Your baby is learning about facial expressions.
- When your baby looks at you, talk or smile back. Use the serve and return method described above.
- Don't worry if your baby doesn't always focus on your face. They need to be in the right mood for face-gazing.
- Do face-to-face play. Recline on a couple pillows and lift your knees. Sit baby on your belly with their back leaning against your thighs (see illustration above).
- When your baby is lying in your lap, softly say their name. Smile or show excitement when your baby turns to you, rewarding your baby for responding.
- Above the crib, place a colorful mobile that is interesting to look at from below. Sometimes mobiles look great from the side but are not very interesting from the baby's view.

Hearing (Zero to two months)

- ☑ I turn my head toward a sound or voice.
- ☑ I prefer human sounds to other sounds.
- ☑ I calm down and listen when you speak to me.
- ☑ I am interested in sounds but sometimes I prefer the quiet.

Hearing Action Plan (Zero to two months)

- Talk and read to your baby. Your baby is learning about language and to recognize your voice.
- Play all kinds of music for your baby. Do not use earbuds or headphones as your baby cannot tell you if it's too loud.
- Protect your baby from loud noises. Noises louder than eighty decibels might cause stress. The decibels generated by a door slamming, thunder, a blender, and so on, are too loud for their sensitive ears. Don't take baby to a sports game, concert, or movie theater.
- Play low-decibel background, or white, noise, such as a fan. This soothes and promotes sleep.

"Talking" (Zero to two months)

- ☑ Crying is how I "talk," or communicate. At first, my cry sounds the same for everything.
- ☑ Near two months corrected age, I make cooing sounds. These sound like vowels: "ahhh," "eeee," "ohhh," "uhhh."
- ☑ I might "talk" with you if you respond to me when I am cooing. We can have a lovely chat!
- ☑ I like to make "yummy" sounds when I feed. This might sound like "mmmm." This means I am enjoying my feed!
- ☑ At the end of this stage, you will hear slight differences in my cry as I learn to communicate. My cry might become louder or more intense for my important needs. It might sound more like fussing for less important needs. My cries for pain, hunger, or boredom sound different.

"Talking" Action Plan (Zero to two months)

- To respond to cries promptly, using a sleep monitor or keeping baby close by in a safe sleeping area during the day because your baby cannot cry very loudly yet. Do not let them sleep in a car seat or on a couch.
- Pick them up when they're crying.

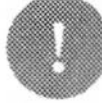

Talk to your baby's doctor if your baby:

- will not stop crying despite you trying to comfort your baby (will not feed, will not quiet down when diaper changed or when held);
- does not turn toward sound or does not startle when there is a loud noise;
- is unable to turn head to the side or cannot lift head briefly in tummy time position at the end of this stage;
- does not have the same movements on both sides of the body.

Two to four months corrected age

I am now two to four months beyond your due date. I have become very familiar with your face and our home. I have learned a lot about how to move my body and make noises. In the next two months, I want to get stronger and learn how to coordinate my arms and legs and become able to communicate better. Will you help me?

Let's look at the developmental skills I will learn from two to four months and the strategies you can use to support me.

Movement (Two to four months)

☑ I actively move my arms and legs when I'm excited. Favorite toys might really get me wiggling.

☑ I love physical play. I love rocking, tickling, touching, bouncing, swinging.

☑ I am learning to move my body and roll a little.

☑ I start to bat at toys if they are close to me when I am lying on my back.

☑ When I lie on my back, I might start to bend my knees and pull them up so my hands can reach them.

☑ I can bring my hands to my chest and face. I might be very good at grabbing your hair or glasses. Sorry about that!

☑ My hands are open, as my grasp reflex has subsided. When I hang on to your finger, you notice that my hands squeeze and relax.

☑ My fingers start to move independently.

☑ I like putting my hands in my mouth.

☑ I like to pat your breast or grasp your skin or clothes when I breastfeed. I like to pat or touch the bottle or grasp your finger when I bottle feed.

☑ I can stand on my legs and feet when you hold me upright. I might like standing on you and practicing leg bends.

☑ At the end of this stage, I can lift my arms and reach for toys that are close to me when I am lying on my back.

Movement Action Plan (Two to four months)

- Play with toys of different shapes, colors, textures, and sounds.
- Encourage rolling from the tummy onto the back. Instead of picking up baby after tummy time, help them roll over and adjust to that feeling. Smile, encourage, and comfort your baby after this movement.
- Allow baby to play on a playmat for longer periods, while baby is content, to support their looking around and learning to roll and reach. Change toys frequently to maintain their interest.
- When baby is on the playmat, ensure hanging toys are within reach. Add extra rings or use bigger toys so your baby can bat at them.
- If baby does not bring hands forward to the middle of their body when sitting in your lap, help move their shoulders forward. When you look down at your baby, their back and shoulders should form the letter "U" (see illustration below).
- Place baby on their side with a big roll behind their back while on the playmat. Alternate sides. Move your baby to a safe sleeping place if they fall asleep. Do not let baby sleep on their side.
- Never leave baby unattended on a bed, couch, or change table, as they may roll and fall off.
- Let baby put their hands in their mouth. Hands are baby's first and best toy. They are learning about their mouth, hand-to-mouth coordination, and self-consoling strategies.
- Move baby's arms and legs to teach them about their body. Play pat-a-cake to music, with their hands or feet.
- Place a small cloth on baby's face to test if they can bring their hands up and remove the cloth.
- After feeds and burping, when baby is relaxed, put them in the crib. This teaches them how to self-console and fall asleep. They will probably need your help more often than not, but it's a good time to start trying.
- If your baby is healthy, consider enrolling in a baby class for playtime.
- At the end of this stage, if your baby cannot lift their arms to bat at toys while on their back, place a rolled-up cloth behind the shoulders to position the shoulders and arms closer to the toys, or move shoulder forward as illustrated below. Your baby learns to use their arms and hands faster if they can see them. We call this the "T. rex" position.

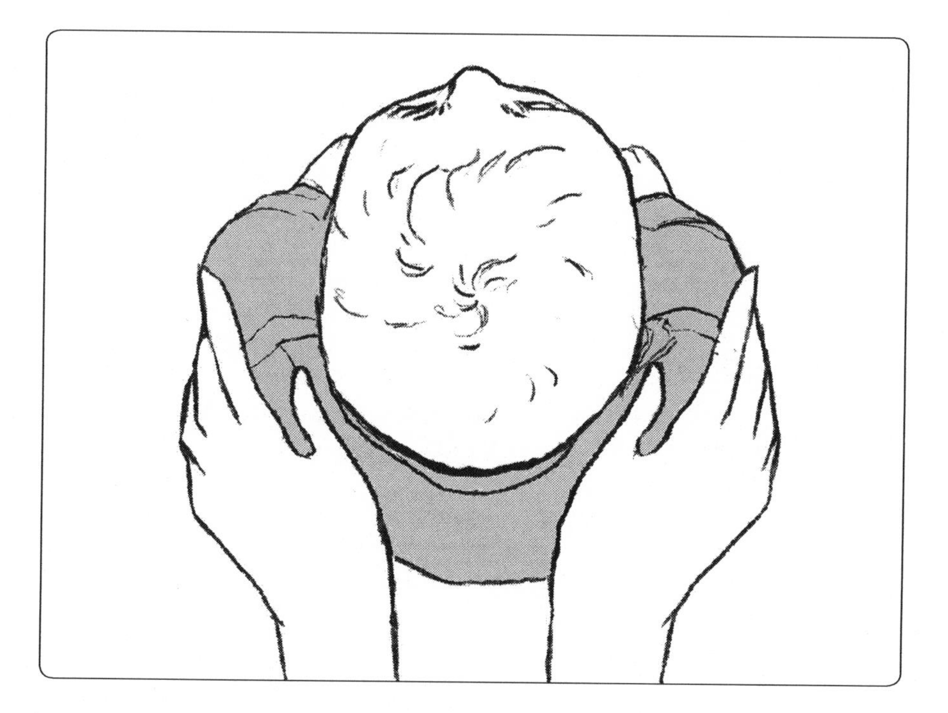

“U” position, with baby’s shoulder and neck gently curved.

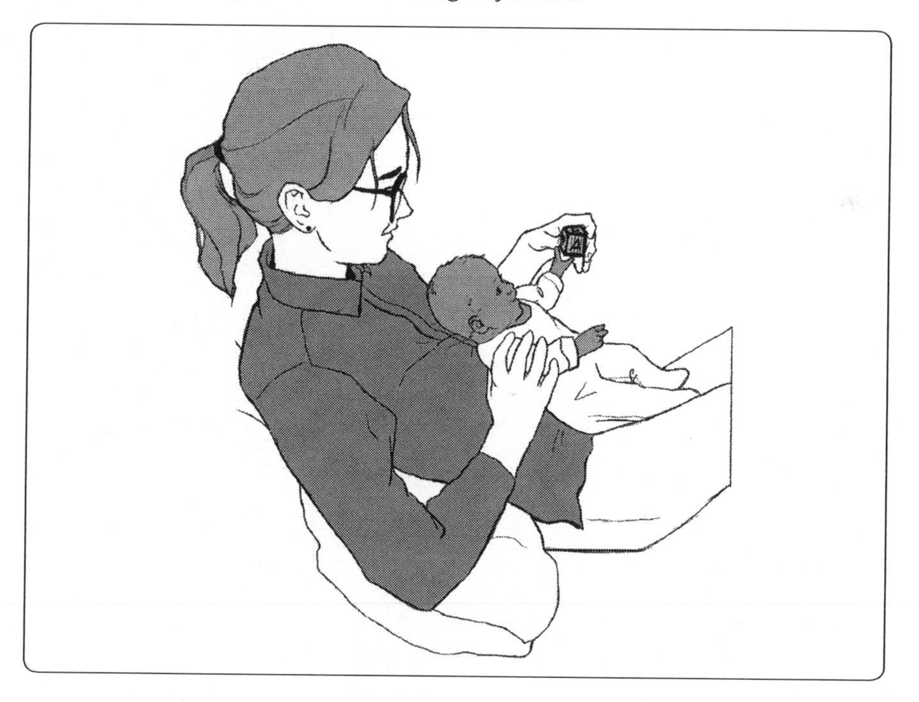

Encouraging “T. rex” positioning of arms.

Behavior (Two to four months)

- ☑ I am awake for longer periods.
- ☑ I am quiet and content when I am not tired or hungry.
- ☑ I am learning how to comfort myself. I might wiggle until I'm comfortable or bring my hands to my face.
- ☑ I am more and more interested in toys and what is around me.
- ☑ I have a short attention span. After ten minutes or so, I'm ready to look at something else.
- ☑ I show off my smiles. These are real smiles, not just gas!
- ☑ I might not like a soother or pacifier as much anymore.
- ☑ I love social play. Talking and playing are becoming my favorite activities.
- ☑ I love looking at myself in the mirror. I am such a cute baby.
- ☑ I start to recognize our daily patterns, such as where you sit at feeding time or where we change my diaper. I like routines and consistency.

Behavior Action Plan (Two to four months)

- Enjoy playtime! Tickle your baby, rub noses, play with their toes and fingers.
- Massage baby to teach them about their body and relax them.
- Ask someone else to help if baby's crying overwhelms you. Never shake baby. If you are alone, put them in a safe place while you take a couple of minutes to relax, then try again to calm them.
- Watch for signs of overstimulation, such as frustration, fussiness, crying, arching, looking away. Stop the activity and give baby some quiet time.
- Don't worry if your baby shows "stranger anxiety." This phase may start around four months and last until baby is more than one year old. Inform others that stranger anxiety is a normal phase. Introduce baby to lots of people while you hold baby. Let people hold baby or be near if baby is calm. Stay close and reassure baby.

Head Control (Two to four months)

- ☑ My head control is stronger now. I can hold my head steadier when I am in a sitting position.
- ☑ I can lift my head between forty-five and ninety degrees during tummy time. I can put weight on my arms to help me lift my head during tummy time.
- ☑ I can briefly lift my head up during tummy time. My chin will be off the floor by about five centimeters (two inches).
- ☑ If I am really good at tummy time, I can lift myself up high and might roll over. If this surprises or frightens me, I might cry.

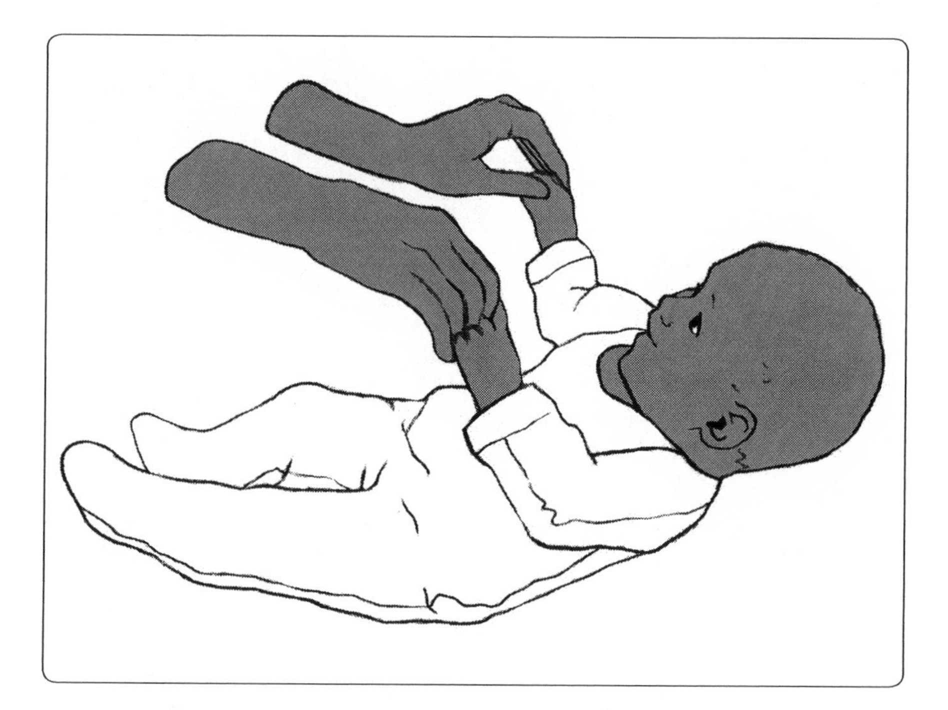

Baby pulling up without head lag.

☑ At the end of this stage, I can lift my head up to ninety degrees during tummy time and look at toys in front of me.

☑ I can keep my head level with my body during airplane exercise. At the end of this stage I can lift my head up to look outward.

☑ At the end of this stage, my head doesn't lag back when I am pulled up from lying down (see illustration above).

Head Control Action Plan (Two to four months)

- Strengthen baby's head control with several tummy time practices a day, lengthen the duration, and use a colorful blanket or mat to stimulate baby's interest. (See tummy time tips above.)
- Practice the airplane exercise. Pretend your baby is flying as "Super Baby" to show them things in the room.
- Practice sitting. If baby's head still bobs, try sitting them on your lap, facing outward so they can look at the room. Once baby has a steady head while sitting, lower your hands down their body to encourage their control of the upper body while seated. Upper body control is essential for sitting in a high chair. Talk to your baby's doctor if your baby always tips to one side.

Vision (Two to four months)

- ☑ I can track faces and toys in all directions. I move my head to watch these. I like to watch moving people.
- ☑ I might stop crying when I see you come near.
- ☑ I might still be cross-eyed at times. I am learning how to focus near and far. This is called "binocular vision."
- ☑ I can see much farther, as far as you can. I like looking at things on the walls and I love ceiling lights or fans.
- ☑ I like looking at patterns.
- ☑ When I see certain toys, I might get very excited.
- ☑ Now that I can raise my hand up, you might see me staring at my hand. It's so amazing!
- ☑ I am starting to develop hand-eye coordination. At the end of this stage, I will try to reach for toys.

Vision Action Plan (Two to four months)

- Place baby in front of a mirror.
- Place a toy in front of baby and slowly move it sideways and up and down. At first, they will track it with eyes only but eventually will learn how to turn their head.
- Teach your baby how to play peekaboo.
- Practice the serve and return pattern of infant behavior development. (See above.)

Hearing (Two to four months)

- ☑ I don't startle at loud noises as much now.
- ☑ I love listening to your voice.
- ☑ When I hear sounds, I turn my eyes to look in the direction they came from. I turn my head, too.
- ☑ When I hear sounds I like, I move my body in excitement.
- ☑ When I hear sounds I don't like, I might show fear or stress.

Hearing Action Plan (Two to four months)

- Read or talk to baby.
- Use an animated or high-pitched voice so baby hears different voice tones.
- Play music, but not too loudly.

"Talking" (Two to four months)

- ☑ I make more sounds now.
- ☑ I like to coo and talk to myself.
- ☑ I love to talk with you.
- ☑ My "talking" reflects my mood. I can sound angry and impatient or happy and playful.
- ☑ I am starting to laugh.
- ☑ I can communicate more clearly now. You are learning to tell if I am hungry or lonely or in pain.
- ☑ I like to squeal. This is a happy, loud sound that I like to try out.
- ☑ I cry or fuss when I'm lonely so that I get some attention.
- ☑ At the end of this stage, when I learn to use the back of my mouth and throat in a new way, I make the sounds of consonants, such as *G*, *K*, or *H*.

"Talking" Action Plan (Two to four months)

- Speak to your baby face-to-face.
- Listen carefully to your baby's cry. It varies for different reasons now (see above).

Talk to your baby's doctor if your baby:

!

- will not stop crying despite your trying to comfort them (will not feed, will not quiet down when diaper changed or when held);
- does not turn toward sound or does not startle when there is a loud noise;
- does not make eye contact;
- does not smile;
- does not follow toys;
- consistently tips head to one side when held in sitting position (cannot keep head midline);
- is not starting to reach;
- has stiff or floppy legs;
- does not stand on feet when held in standing position;
- does not have the same movements on both sides of the body;
- is unable to hold head ninety degrees from tummy time position at the end of this stage.

Four to six months corrected age

Wow! I am now four to six months beyond your due date.

I have become a busy baby. My head control is stronger and I'm discovering how my body works. I am also learning to communicate better, so you understand what I need. In the next two months I want to figure out how to use my arms. Let's play together!

Let's look at the developmental skills I will learn from four to six months and the strategies you can use to support me.

Movement (Four to six months)

- ☑ I like to spend more time on a playmat. I learn a lot about my body and my environment when I'm on the floor.
- ☑ I get up high during tummy time, and I can roll from my tummy onto my back. This is a big roll for me!
- ☑ I can move myself to a different location and position when I'm left on my tummy or back. Always be sure I'm left in a safe place.
- ☑ I am working on rolling from lying on my back to lying on my tummy. This is hard work. I might roll my hips first or I might try to roll my arms and shoulders over first. It doesn't matter how I roll, as long as I figure out what works for me.
- ☑ My reach is becoming more accurate. I use the palm of my hand to grasp objects.
- ☑ I am able to use my fingers separately. These are my fiddling fingers and I'll get them caught in your hair or in your necklace. I might pinch you, sorry!
- ☑ I reach for my image in a mirror.
- ☑ I can put my fingers and toys in my mouth. Sometimes I put my hand a little too far inside my mouth. Oops! I learn that makes me gag.
- ☑ When I have a toy in each hand, I can bang them together.
- ☑ When I'm on my tummy, I can reach for and play with toys.
- ☑ When I am lying on my back and you pull me up by my hands, my head comes up, either with my body or when I do a little tummy crunch and pull my head up first.

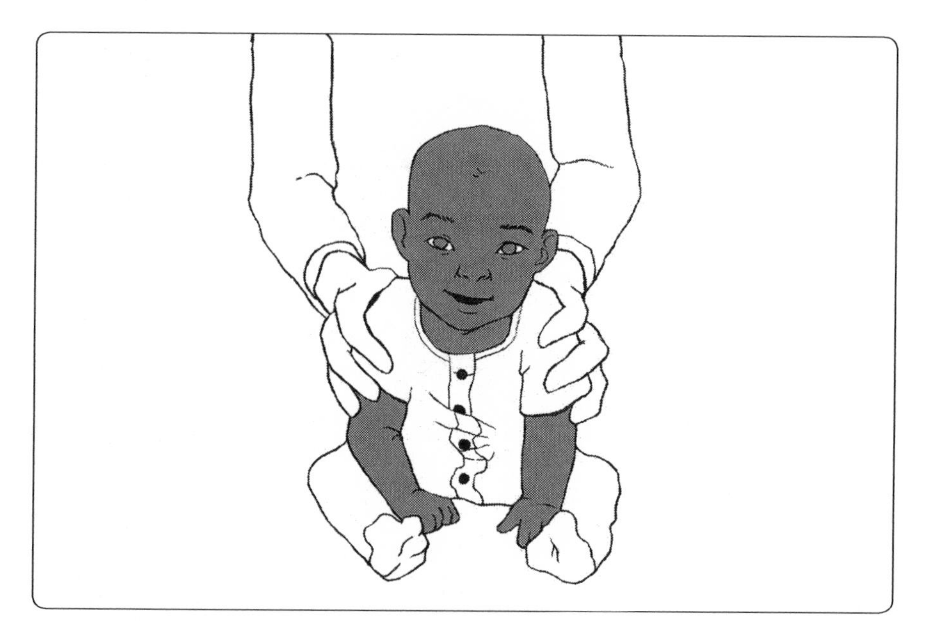

Tripod sitting.

☑ When I'm lying on my back, I might reach for my toes. Sometimes, I can pull my toes all the way into my mouth. Can you do that, Mom or Dad?

☑ I can stand with your help. You don't need to support me as much as before.

☑ When I'm standing, I like to bounce up and down.

☑ At the end of this stage, I start to reach out to you when I want to be picked up. You won't be able to resist me.

☑ At the end of this stage, I not only look for dropped objects, but I also reach to pick them up again. I'm so smart.

☑ At the end of this stage, I can do a "tripod sit" (see illustration above). My hands keep me from falling over.

Movement Action Plan (Four to six months)

- Let baby spend awake time on their back on a playmat with colorful toys suspended overhead but within reach. Place toys beside baby so they can look around. Change the toys regularly to keep your baby's interest.
- Lay baby on their back and pull them up by the hands (see illustration below). You might feel them pulling up as well. Tummy crunches are good work for baby. If their head lags, practice tummy crunches more often.

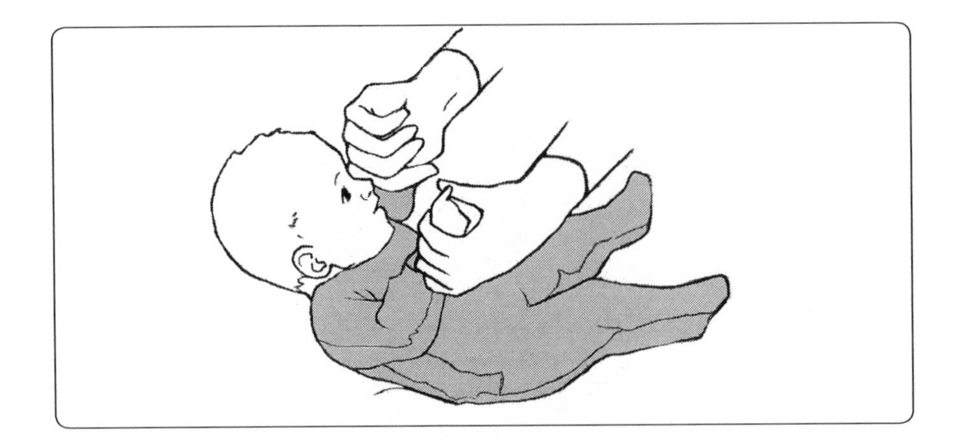

Practice tummy crunches with baby.

- Make tummy time more challenging for baby by placing a toy in front of their head. They might face-plant, so be sure the blanket is soft. With practice, your baby will learn how to reach while doing tummy time. At this age, your baby should spend close to an hour total each day in tummy time.
- When tummy time is over, roll baby onto their back. This is a good rehearsal for babies to eventually do by themselves.
- Put baby in a recliner chair so they can sit up and watch household activity. Avoid long periods in the recliner, which may cause flattening of the back of the head. (See chapter 3.)
- Always buckle your baby into their bouncy chair, swing, or stroller to avoid the risk of falling.
- When baby can sit without support, lower the crib mattress, because before long baby will pull up to standing.
- Give baby toys that are safe to hold and put in their mouth.
- Let your baby touch different textures: a soft furry teddy bear, a hard ball, a rough cloth, a bumpy toy.
- Try the “trade” game. Give your baby a toy to hold and then offer their favorite toy. Can they figure out how to drop the first toy?
- Offer a toy for each hand and encourage baby to bang them together. Toys that make noise are best. Look happy and sound excited when your baby bangs the toys together.
- Support baby when they stand and bounce. If your baby grips the ground with their toes when standing, support some of their body weight and allow standing for a short time only. This is the newborn toe-grasp reflex and it will subside soon. Standing for long periods with this reflex will make your baby’s leg muscles develop incorrectly and affect how they walk and run. At this age,

do not use baby equipment in which baby stands for long periods, such as Jolly Jumpers or exersaucers.

Behavior (Four to six months)

- ☑ I can imitate your facial expression. I'm like a mirror.
- ☑ I smile at you if you have a happy expression or talk to me in a pleasant voice.
- ☑ I get upset or scared if you have an unhappy face or talk to me in an angry voice.
- ☑ I communicate my likes and dislikes.
- ☑ I show an angry or upset face if you take away something I really like.
- ☑ I can have moods and can change them quickly.
- ☑ I might quiet down when I hear music or sounds.
- ☑ I show excitement when you come to me. Yay, you're here!
- ☑ I might like to hang out with people and watch and listen to them.
- ☑ I may show stranger anxiety when I see someone I don't know. I might look scared, I might cry, or I might not be as friendly as I usually am.
- ☑ I might have favorite toys or objects that I like to look at. These might make me happy or help me calm down.

Behavior Action Plan (Four to six months)

- Know your baby's limits. Their temperament is emerging now and their behavior will indicate likes and dislikes, how long they can pay attention, and how easily they are calmed.
- Make sleep-time routines consistent. You might start with massage and end with singing while sitting in a chair in baby's bedroom with dimmed lights. Routines will help your baby recognize the steps toward sleep.
- Allow baby to watch you when you eat. They are not ready for solids yet, but can learn about the spoon while watching you use yours. Keep an empty baby spoon nearby and pretend to feed baby. Touch baby's lips with the dry baby spoon. If they open their mouth, put the spoon in their mouth and let them get to know it. Your baby will be ready for solids near six months corrected age.
- To stimulate interest, provide toys that change when touched or moved, such one that lights up, plays a tune, or has moving parts inside.
- Show your baby a toy and then cover it with a blanket. Can your baby figure out how to find the toy? At this age your baby is starting to learn about object permanence. It will take your baby a few months to figure out this game.
- Get out together. Try rides in a stroller and visiting different places and people.
- Remember that stranger anxiety may last until baby is more than one year old. Continue to introduce baby to lots of people, at first holding baby while

in the presence of other people, then progressing to other people holding them while you are nearby.

Head Control (Four to six months)

- ☑ I can hold my head steady and in midline when I am in a sitting position.
- ☑ I can lift my head ninety degrees during tummy time. I can put weight on my arms to help my head lift be stronger. I can push myself up so far that my elbows are off the floor and I'm almost on my hands.

Head Control Action Plan (Four to six months)

- Try baby chairs, such as those made by Bumbo, only if baby can keep their body straight. It's not good for your baby to sit for long periods when tipped to one side or if their head keeps falling forward.
- Try a high chair if baby can keep their head straight in a seated position. Some high chairs tip back slightly to make control of the head and upper body easier. If the high chair is too large for baby, buckle them into the chair and add big rolls around their sides. While they're in the high chair, always watch baby to prevent them from slipping out or tipping forward or sideways. If, with the rolls, the high chair is still too big for baby, put it aside for a couple weeks or months.

Vision (Four to six months)

- ☑ I am more aware of my environment and I'll look around and notice objects and people.
- ☑ I can track a moving object or person with my eyes.
- ☑ I still love to look at myself in a mirror.
- ☑ I like to look at my hands when I'm lying on my back.
- ☑ I like brightly colored toys.
- ☑ If I am sitting with you and I drop a toy, I look for the toy. I am figuring out gravity.
- ☑ My hand-eye coordination is getting so good. You'll see me try to line up my hand and fingers to reach and grasp a toy. Sometimes I'll miss, but I'll get better.
- ☑ At the end of this stage, my eyes do not cross anymore. My eyes move simultaneously when I am looking up and down, sideways, and near and far.

Vision Action Plan (Four to six months)

- Make it a game for baby to mimic your facial expressions. Smile, frown, or look surprised.

- Try this funny face game: Show your face to baby and then put something different on your face, such a sticker, clown nose, or funny glasses. Do they notice something different and reach up to touch that new thing?
- Play peekaboo. Hold a book in front of your baby and call your baby's name. See if your baby knows to look around the book to find you.
- Play "dropsy" with your baby. Show your baby a toy and then let it fall. Can your baby figure out where it went? Keep practicing this with your baby.
- Sit your baby in front of a mirror. They might start reaching for the mirror.
- Book your baby for a routine eye exam around six months corrected age.

Hearing (Four to six months)

☑ I like to hear you talk, sing, hum, or read out loud.
☑ When I hear a sound, I turn my head and look in that direction.
☑ When I hear your quiet voice, I might calm down.
☑ When I hear loud, sudden noises, I might get frightened.

Hearing Action Plan (Four to six months)

- Sing during activities and read to your baby every day.
- Play music. Your baby does not need television time at this age.

"Talking" (Four to six months)

☑ I squeal with delight when I'm very excited.
☑ I can imitate sounds.
☑ I babble more and more. I like hearing myself.
☑ My cry can rise and fall in tone. When I am very upset, I can make my cry intensify.
☑ I might cry or fuss when I'm bored or lonely. Where are you? Can you come play?
☑ I can really project my voice if I need something.
☑ I can communicate that I like some things and not others.
☑ I make sounds to communicate my displeasure if my toys are taken away.
☑ I can laugh out loud.
☑ I can make two-syllable sounds, such as "ah-goo."

"Talking" Action Plan (Four to six months)

- Talk with your baby. Say something and then wait for your baby to respond. You'll have a conversation that will make no sense, but is a wonderful opportunity for baby to learn about language and talking.

Talk to your baby's doctor if your baby:

- cannot lift their head from tummy time;
- has a head that lags back when working on tummy crunches;
- does not stand on feet when held in standing position;
- does not have the same movements on both sides of the body;
- has not started rolling;
- is cross-eyed;
- does not look at things around them;
- is not starting to reach for toys when lying on back;
- can only reach with one hand;
- cannot bring hands to mouth;
- cannot hold a toy;
- does not sit with support;
- does not make babbling sounds;
- does not turn toward sound;
- does not smile;
- has stiff or floppy legs;
- cannot sit in a tripod position or with support at six months corrected age.

Six to nine months corrected age

I'm already six to nine months beyond your due date. I am very curious about my world. I like toys and fun activities. Now I can put anything in my mouth, so you need to keep my area free of choking hazards and yucky stuff. Dust bunnies are interesting but not good for me. I want to learn how to communicate better and how to sit and crawl.

The following table shows the developmental skills I will learn from six to nine months and the strategies you can use to support me.

Movement (Six to nine months)

- ☑ I will reach my hands out to you to pick me up.
- ☑ I can wave "bye-bye."
- ☑ I hold on to Mom's breast or a bottle during feeding.
- ☑ I can roll from tummy time to my back.
- ☑ I can roll from my back to my tummy.
- ☑ I can sit with pillow support and eventually by myself.
- ☑ I can push up to my hands and knees and rock in place (see illustration below).

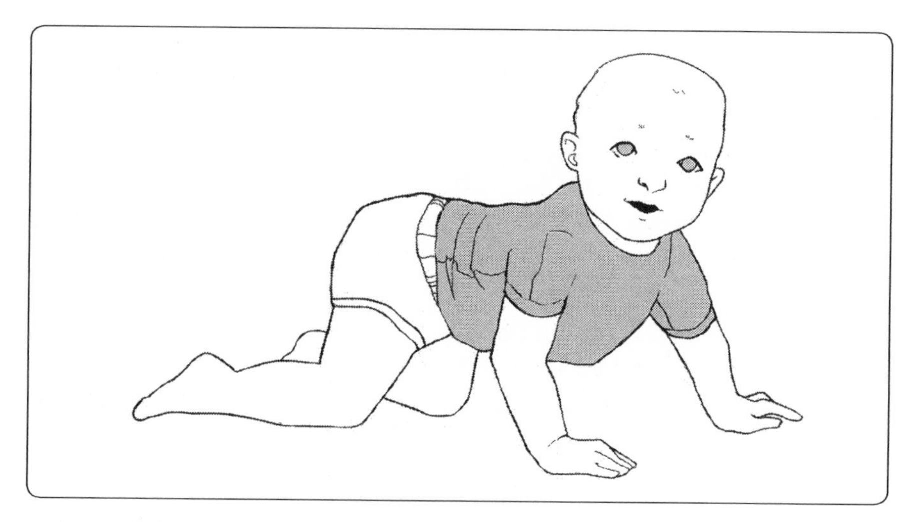

Push up to hands and knees.

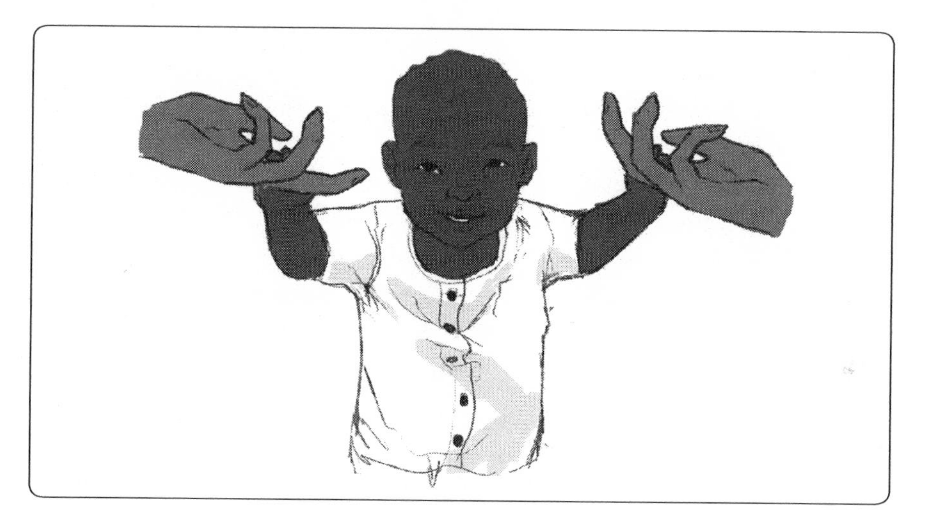

Pull up to standing.

- ☑ I can pull myself to standing if I hang on to your hands or a finger (see illustration above).
- ☑ I can stand on my legs with very little support from you.
- ☑ My finger accuracy is improving, and I can pick up small toys or small pieces of food.
- ☑ Everything I pick up ends up in my mouth. Beware.
- ☑ I can transfer a toy from one hand to the other.
- ☑ At the end of this stage, I can stand for a while when holding on to the couch or coffee table.

☑ At the end of this stage I can crawl forward, perhaps with my stomach on the floor. I might even figure out how to crawl backward first. There are no wrong ways to crawl!

Movement Action Plan (Six to nine months)

- Childproof your home. Baby can move about and put things in their mouth. Add gates on the stairs, locks on cupboards, covers on electrical outlets, and remove things your baby can choke on.
- If baby is big enough, try placing them in an outdoor swing. Ensure your baby will not fall through the leg hole. Gently push baby in the swing. Can they maintain head control? Are they relaxed or afraid? Reassure baby and slow down or stop if they act scared.
- Remove the mobile from the crib when baby is ready to stand on their own. They could really hurt themselves if they grabbed the mobile and fell.
- Play outside. Use sunscreen or bug repellant on baby's skin but choose safe products.
- Play pat-a-cake with baby in your lap facing away from you. Hold their hands and move them while you sing. Practice this with baby facing you, in a bouncy chair so they can feel the action, listen to your voice, and watch your animated face (see illustration below).
- Try the "trade" game. (See description in four- to six-month section above.)
- Be sure all objects within baby's reach are baby-safe.
- Rotate baby's toys regularly. After a few days hidden, toys that reemerge will be new and exciting.
- Continue giving baby different textures to touch and play with.
- Give baby toys to shake or bang together. A wooden spoon and upside-down pot will be really fun.
- Put toys inside a container and let baby discover them. Teach baby how to put toys inside the container.
- Stack toys and make them fall down.
- Blow bubbles nearby so baby can reach for them.
- Sit opposite baby and roll a ball toward them, teaching them how to roll it back to you. This is difficult.
- Continue tummy time. Place toys out of baby's reach to encourage baby to move or crawl to them.
- Play on the floor. Baby will build muscle coordination and strength better on the floor than sitting in baby equipment.
- Lay on the floor and let baby crawl all over you. Do stretches together.
- Always strap your baby into their high chair, swing, bouncy chair, or stroller.

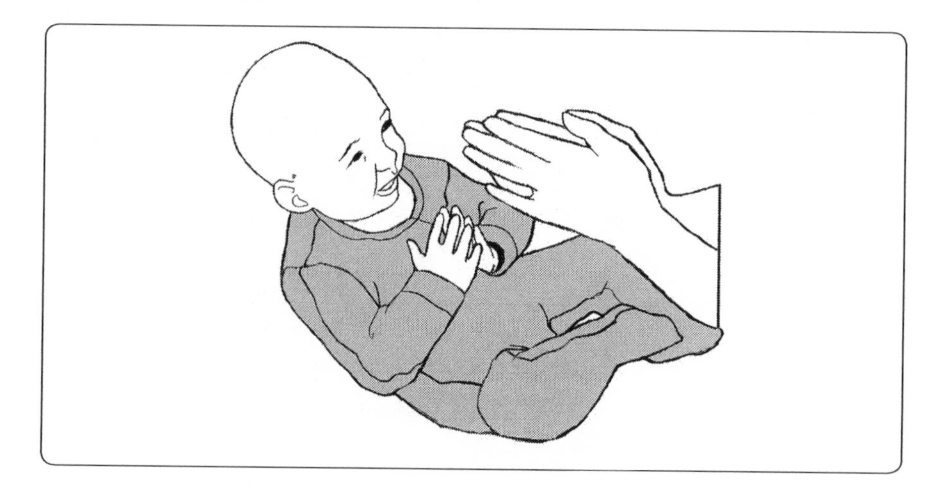

Play pat-a-cake with baby.

Behavior (Six to nine months)

- ☑ My personality is emerging. Do I tend to be quiet, active, shy, social? Do I approach new activities cautiously or eagerly?
- ☑ I like playing peekaboo!
- ☑ I look for toys after they disappear from my sight. For example, when a toy is covered up with a blanket, I look for it. If it is dropped, I look down for it. This is called the development of object permanence. I know the toy still exists even when I can't see it.
- ☑ I complain if you take something I like away from me or if you stop doing something I like. I can be very demanding.
- ☑ If you ask me, "Where is Mama?" I turn my head and look for Mom.
- ☑ My attention span is lengthening. I can entertain myself with toys for a little while.

Behavior Action Plan (Six to nine months)

- Get to know baby's personality to learn how to best support them. If baby tends to be cautious, let your baby warm up to new areas. If your baby is shy, provide reassurance when meeting new people, and so on.
- When baby makes noises (crying or fussing), talk to them while you get what you think they need. If you can't get to baby right away, reassure them that you hear and are coming. Tell baby what you need to do, such as warm up their food or wash the toy.
- If baby expresses frustration because they can't do something, help problem-solve. Maybe they need a boost to get closer or help getting out of an uncomfortable position. Tell them what you are doing to help.

- If baby is cranky, reduce stimulation so that they regain self-control. Sometimes they want to be held; sometimes they need to be by themselves.
- Continue baby massage.
- If your baby still has stranger anxiety or fear of new places, give verbal reassurance. Keep exposing your baby to new people and places.
- Establish routines for baby's security. Routines before naps and night sleep are particularly important. Your baby will learn what happens next and will become better at relaxing to sleep. Lay your baby down before they are fully asleep so that they learn how to put themselves to sleep.
- Move baby's crib to their own room. Ensure you can hear baby cry from your bedroom. If not, use a baby monitor. This transition may be hard on you both. Your baby will need reassurance.

Head Control (Six to nine months)

- ☑ My head control is steady when I'm sitting, standing, or being held.
- ☑ From tummy time, I easily lift my head and shoulders up.

Head Control Action Plan (Six to nine months)

- If your baby can keep their head and upper body steady in sitting position, sit them in high chairs or baby chairs.
- If your baby's head tips to the side or forward, stop doing play time in sitting position. Your baby might need a little roll beside them to help keep straight.

Vision (Six to nine months)

- ☑ I can now see all colors.
- ☑ I enjoy seeing toys with different shapes, colors, and patterns.
- ☑ I am interested in picture books.
- ☑ I am learning to recognize facial expressions, such as happiness, anger, sadness.
- ☑ I watch you closely and imitate your actions.

Vision Action Plan (Six to nine months)

- Show your baby picture books and point out the pictures.

Hearing (Six to nine months)

- ☑ I am learning the meaning of various words, such as "mama," "dada," "dog," and "no."
- ☑ When I hear my name, I turn my head. I like it when you call me by name.

- [x] I am starting to understand different tones of voice, like when you are happy or angry.
- [x] I am starting to understand simple directions, such as "come here."

Hearing Action Plan (Six to nine months)

- Know that at more than six months old, baby's ears can differentiate the sounds of language. They're listening very carefully to your words and how you speak. They may try to mimic you.
- Continue reading to baby daily so they can hear the sounds of your language(s).
- Use baby's name when you want their attention.

"Talking" (Six to nine months)

- [x] I copy sounds that you make. If I hear you cough, I might cough, too. If you laugh, I will probably join you (even if I didn't understand the joke).
- [x] I like to stick out my tongue and make "raspberries."
- [x] I am learning to make different sounds, such as "ch," "bl," "da," "ga."
- [x] I can voice words, such as "baba," "mama," "dada."
- [x] I can imitate animal sounds, such as "woof woof," "baa baa," "meow."
- [x] I can change the tone of my voice to convey whether I am happy or unhappy.

"Talking" Action Plan (Six to nine months)

- Talk and sing with your baby.
- Tell your baby what you are doing when you are caring for them. Describe the clothes you are putting on your baby, talk about their bath, describe their food, the weather. Any conversation is great.

Talk to your baby's doctor if your baby:

- cannot stand on two feet while you hold their hands;
- does not have the same movements on both sides of the body;
- cannot lift upper body from tummy time;
- does not sit in tripod position (arms helping stay in seated position);
- cannot hold head steady or in midline when sitting;
- cannot pick up a toy with one hand;
- cannot bring hands, toys, or food to mouth;
- has not started to sit with minimal support;
- does not respond when called;
- does not look around the room at objects and people;

- is cross-eyed;
- does not make sounds;
- does not laugh or squeal (make loud noises).

Nine to twelve months corrected age

Look at me! I am nine to twelve months beyond your due date. I love to explore. I can move around my world and get into all sorts of trouble. I can entertain myself for longer periods of time. I'm learning to make and understand words and I can even grasp a few simple commands. My big task in this stage is getting ready to stand by myself.

The following table shows the developmental skills I will learn from nine to twelve months and the strategies you can use to support me.

Movement (Nine to twelve months)

- ☑ I can crawl frontward or backward.
- ☑ I can pull myself up to a sitting position.
- ☑ I can sit by myself for a little while.
- ☑ I can turn around in a circle when I'm sitting.
- ☑ I like to wiggle and dance to music. Hang on to my fingers or I'll topple over!
- ☑ I start to walk while holding on to your finger or the furniture.
- ☑ I am learning how to climb up and down stairs. I usually do this on my knees. I'm not very good at this yet.
- ☑ I can help a little when you are trying to dress me. For example, I can hold out my leg when you pull up my pants.
- ☑ I like to play pat-a-cake and clap my hands together.
- ☑ I like to feed myself, although I am very messy. I'm better with my hands and am learning how to get the spoon into my mouth.
- ☑ I can drink from a cup.
- ☑ I can pick up a toy and hold it between my fingers and thumb (called "pincher grasp").
- ☑ I can transfer a toy from one container and to another.
- ☑ I can give you a toy if you ask me. Ask me nicely and I might comply.
- ☑ I can move a toy from one hand to my other hand.
- ☑ I like to splash water. Sorry I'm making you wet during my bath.
- ☑ I can throw a ball. Please pick it up for me and let the game begin!

- ☑ I can turn the pages of a book. Board books are better for me so I don't tear the pages.
- ☑ At the end of this stage, I can pull myself to standing.
- ☑ At the end of this stage, I can stand by myself for a short time. I am wobbly at first.

Movement Action Plan (Nine to twelve months)

- Give your baby safe toys in a safe place. Change toys regularly so baby gets excited for every playtime. Playing is how baby learns.
- Let your baby lead playtime activities. Throwing toys around might be their fun game today. Or dropping toys and making you pick them up. Your baby will make a new game out of any safe object, such as a wooden spoon or telephone.
- Stack up toys until they fall. Be excited when the toys fall down.
- Entertain your baby by filling a box with an assortment of toys, baby books, plastic containers, teddy bears, and let your baby explore what's inside the box.
- Give baby toys that make a noise when shaken or banged together. A tambourine might be fun. How about a toy that pops up or changes when you manipulate it?
- Play pat-a-cake facing one another.
- Chase and tickle your baby. Physical play is fun.
- Take the airplane exercise up a level. Can you "fly" your baby toward a toy and ask them to pick it up? This requires great strength and coordination for baby.
- Dance to music.
- Roll toys away or point at toys and encourage baby to fetch them. Let your baby be creative in how to get there. If they're able to stand, hold their hands to walk over to the toy. Let baby figure out how to bend down to get it.
- Make an obstacle course with pillows and toys. Can your baby figure out how to get to you through the obstacle course?
- Help your baby learn how to climb up and down stairs. Be ready to support and catch baby. Block the stairs afterward so baby can't access them.
- Play outside.
- Let baby splash in water—but always supervise. Baby could fall into and drown in only two inches of water.
- Register for swim playtime for babies. Pools with a warmer water are more pleasant.
- Always strap your baby into baby equipment, such as high chairs, strollers, swings, as they can fall very easily.

Behavior (Nine to twelve months)

- ☑ My attention span continues to lengthen and playtime lasts longer before I become bored or tired of it.
- ☑ I imitate your actions, such as putting a phone to my ear, feeding myself, holding a tissue to my nose, hugging or kissing a doll or teddy bear.
- ☑ I understand simple phrases, like "up," "no," and "all gone." That "no" word is not my favorite.
- ☑ If you laugh or express joy at something I do, I repeat it over and over again.
- ☑ I can drop a toy or give you a toy if you ask. But maybe not my favorite toy!
- ☑ I show signs of emotions, such as happiness, affection, fear, or jealousy.
- ☑ I might still show stranger anxiety and might show fear when I'm in a new place. I will look to you for reassurance. It will help me relax if I see you are not afraid.
- ☑ I might cry if I have pulled myself up to standing but I'm tired and I don't know how to sit down by myself. Help!

Behavior Action Plan (Nine to twelve months)

- Follow daytime routines. Baby likes routines for play, reading, feeding, bathing, and napping. When these routines are disrupted, such as during travel, baby may be unsettled and need reassurance from you.
- Follow bedtime routines so that baby understands bedtime and feels secure. Sleeping in their own room might still be hard. Continue reassuring. If baby has to sleep in a new place, they may not sleep as well at first.
- Continue to learn about baby's personality. Talk to baby about how you think they're feeling. Use words to describe their mood, for example, saying, "You sure are happy today." Or "You look tired." If your baby is moody, give them a safe, quiet place to relax.
- Give your baby choices: "Do you want the blue shirt or the green shirt?" "Do you want to eat carrots or peas?"
- Let baby explore safe toys and environments.
- Spend time and be playful with your baby.
- Know that stranger anxiety should be easing now. Continue exposing baby to new people and things. Baby watches your reaction. If you appear afraid or worried, baby will be more anxious. It will help baby relax if they see you are not afraid. Smile and be encouraging.
- Let your baby be curious about food and get really, really messy. Take off their shirt before you feed them. Clean up baby after the meal.

Vision (Nine to twelve months)

☑ I like imitating facial expressions.
☑ My hand-eye coordination is improving, and I can reach quite accurately.
☑ I can follow quickly moving objects

Vision Action Plan (Nine to twelve months)

- Sit baby in your lap with a book and point out objects, colors, and shapes. Ask your baby to find items in the book. "Where's the red ball?"
- Ask your baby to find items in your home. "Where's your green truck?"
- Point out objects in the distance when outside with your baby. "Look, a bird."

Hearing (Nine to twelve months)

☑ I recognize my own name.
☑ I will listen when you talk to me.
☑ I will respond to new sounds.
☑ I will hear quiet sounds if I hold still and quiet!

Hearing Action Plan (Nine to twelve months)

- Continue reading to baby daily. Read with an animated voice. Use different voices for the characters, such as a high-pitched voice for Little Red Riding Hood and a deep voice for the wolf. Point at animal pictures and make animal sounds together.
- Use your baby's name when seeking their attention.

"Talking" (Nine to twelve months)

☑ I can use the words "mama" and "dada" when referring to you.
☑ I like to sing along with you, even if I can't say the words exactly right!
☑ Imitating sounds is still one of my favorite activities with you.
☑ I use my voice to get what I want. I raise my voice or sound angry if I don't get I want. How can you refuse me?

"Talking" Action Plan (Nine to twelve months)

- Name the things in your baby's environment. Point and say the words, such as "dog," "shoes," "book," "tree," "car." Describe the characteristics of objects, such as "soft bear," "bumpy toy," "wet cloth."
- Describe your daily activities to baby.
- Don't use baby talk anymore, as your baby needs to learn language. Use short commands or sentences: "Are you hungry?" "Where's Daddy?" "Don't touch."
- Model good manners when you are with baby. Say thank you and please. Your baby is listening.

Talk to your baby's doctor if your baby:

- is not sitting independently;
- is not crawling;
- is unable to pull to standing when hanging on to your hands;
- cannot stand by without help;
- stands on toes;
- cannot bounce up and down slightly when standing (make little knee bends);
- cannot pick up small toys or pieces of food;
- does not have the same movements on both sides of the body;
- does not imitate sounds;
- does not use single words with meaning, for example "mama" or "dada";
- avoids eye contact;
- is not interested in playing or reading;
- is not watching activities around them.

Developmental milestones beyond one year may be accessed from many resources. Your baby's doctor may have recommendations. Also visit our website at www.preemiecare.ca for suggested resources.

Final Thoughts

You will build a strong parent-baby relationship by learning how your baby communicates and relates to the world. You can foster optimal development through play and stimulating exercises. Have fun with your baby.

Babies grow and develop so quickly. In a heartbeat, your baby is sitting by herself, and then walking, and then in no time at all, she's heading off to school. My advice to other parents is to ENJOY EVERY MOMENT. Don't be in a rush for the next developmental step. Don't always be working on the next task. Don't live for the future. Live today. It's okay to just plunk down with your baby and play with a toy for as long as they want. Make everyday routines into something fun. If you are folding clothes, dump them on the floor and let your baby pick out which one to fold next. If you are cleaning the floor, put on music and dance. Don't sit in front of your baby with a camera stuck to your face all the time. Take one picture and then be present with your baby. These are the moments that you'll cherish.

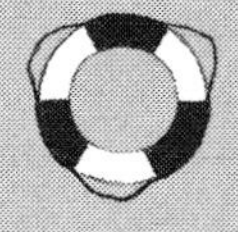

EXPERT TIPS

Here are the key strategies to navigate the journey

- Get to know your baby's unique temperament.
- Get to know your baby's cues.
- Develop your baby's brain through serve and return activities.
- Practice tummy time, a key foundational skill for your baby.
- Learn to discern the characteristics of your baby's cry.
- Try our strategies to calm your fussy or crying baby.
- Know your baby's corrected age.
- Use the developmental checklists to monitor your baby's development.
- Try the action plans to encourage your baby's development.
- If your baby is not keeping up with development despite your work on the action plan or if you have any development concerns, speak to your baby's doctor.

7

KEEPING YOUR HEAD ABOVE WATER
Caring for Yourself

SO MANY parents neglect their personal needs while caring for a premature baby. We know a premature baby involves a lot more work, responsibility, and worry for parents compared with a full-term baby. Parents of premature babies will sacrifice so much to ensure their baby does well. There is no question that the center of attention after NICU discharge is on the baby. But former NICU parents will tell you that you need to take care of yourself, too. Neglecting yourself long-term is not sustainable and carries physical and mental health risks for yourself, your baby, and your family.

In this chapter, we focus on caring for yourself once your baby has been discharged. We reflected on the strategies used by the most successful and happy parents in our practices, those who were able to find that balance between the baby's needs and everyone and everything else. We studied the literature to identify practical ways for parents to be resilient amid high family demands. We provide ideas to keep your life and family balanced. Our six key points serve as your "life preserver" to keep you afloat as you navigate the first year with your baby. In addition, we review the mental health concerns that may develop if your life preserver is not enough. And finally, we close with the place we hope every parent reaches—where you consider life to be "normal" again and you find meaning in your experience of having a premature baby.

Every parent will try to do it all and the best they can. Take care of baby, home, older kids. I think I did a good job with my first, but that baby was full-term. Then came baby number two, a long NICU stay, and home with a premature baby on oxygen. I was stronger physically when I took him home because it had been months since I gave birth. But I wasn't prepared for how exhausting it would be to look after a preemie, go to all those appointments, pump breast milk, work on bottle and breastfeeding, and try to manage reflux. My older child was raised by the television and fast food. We all felt strained and on edge. My partner and I barely spoke to one another. I did not feel healthy or like myself mentally. I started to have flashbacks of the NICU. My baby's nurse asked me how I was doing and I broke into tears. I didn't know where to start to get my life and my family back on track. I'm a very competent person yet I did not see that I should not have neglected my own needs for so long. My gas tank was empty.

Build Your Life Preserver

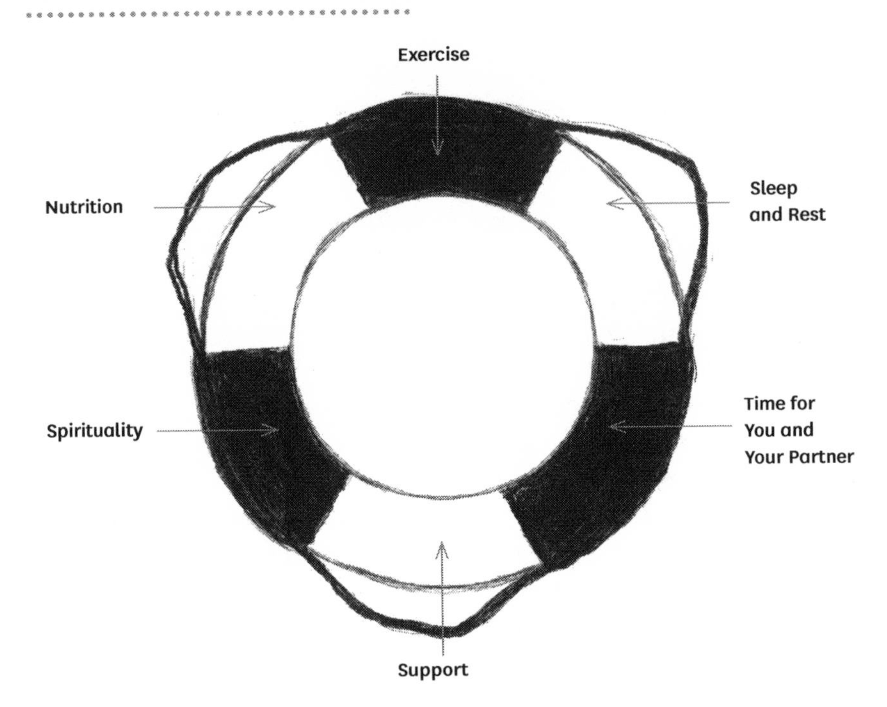

There are six key areas that will help you stay afloat.

Making small changes to improve self-care is one of the first and most important steps you can take to mental and physical wellness. Looking after yourself is key to preventing caregiver burnout. Self-care is important for both mothers and fathers. This section provides you with information on key areas of self-care and suggestions for changes you can make in your life. For you to stay afloat, six key areas require attention.

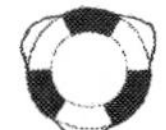

Nutrition

You've made it through the whirlwind experience of the NICU. Hopefully, our tips from chapter 1 helped you look after yourself and know the important role of nutrition in self-care. Now that you are home, you are totally responsible for the care of your preterm baby as well as yourself. It can be difficult to eat well. You may not feel hungry or you may find that you eat mostly unhealthy, convenient foods. Eating nutritious foods regularly throughout the day will help you to feel better and carry on with your daily activities.

> *I remember looking at my husband and breaking into tears when he came in the door after work. All we had for dinner was popcorn. There were no groceries in the house. I was living on coffee and rice cakes. We looked at one another and realized something needed to change. If we were going to care for this preemie and ourselves, we needed better meal-planning and organization around food and nourishment.*

You can make positive changes in your eating habits.

ACTION PLAN: Boosting Your Nutrition

Try these strategies to boost your nutrition:

- Try meal-planning. Sit down with someone who can help with meals. Plan simple meals for the next three to four days at a time. Prepare a shopping list and arrange to get the food items you need. If you have the financial flexibility, use a meal service provider. Even two to three days a week can make a big difference.

- Keep a filled water bottle with you as you move around the house. Satisfy your thirst with milk, beverages fortified with vitamins and minerals, water, and juice. Enjoy caffeinated beverages in moderation. These could affect your baby's sleep and cause irritability if you are breastfeeding or pumping.
- Eat healthy snacks from the four food groups (grains, protein, fruits and vegetables, and dairy) every two hours. Six smaller meals a day may work better for you.
- Prepare for being out of the house. Take a water bottle and packable items, such as fresh fruit, crackers, granola, cheese sticks, protein bars, or nuts so that you have healthy foods on hand while you are out.
- Buy prepared veggies (baby carrots, cherry tomatoes, bagged salad, fresh or dried fruit).
- Choose healthy, easily prepared grains (brown rice, whole wheat pasta, quinoa, whole wheat wraps or tortillas, pita bread and whole grain or rice crackers).
- Drink milk, fortified soy beverage, almond milk, whey protein shakes, Greek yogurt (has more protein), cottage cheese.
- Buy easily prepared meat and alternatives: canned and frozen fish, frozen meat patties, meatballs (turkey or beef), canned lentils, bean and pea soups, frozen meals.
- Make meal preparation manageable. Divide the task of meal-making into small jobs rather than doing it all at once. Chop veggies in the morning, marinate the meat at lunch, and peel potatoes in the afternoon.
- Use a slow cooker for make-ahead meals. The ingredients can be prepared the night before and then simply put in the pot to cook throughout the day.
- Accept offers from others to drop off or make you a meal. Don't forget to ask for meals from your support people. Flowers might be nice, but a meal is sustaining.

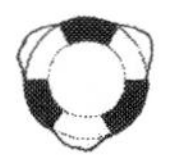

Exercise

Exercise may be difficult to fit into your day or may be the last thing you want to do. However, even a small amount can help. Exercising can actually increase your energy. You just need to take that first step.

> *Returning to exercise was challenging for me. During my pregnancy I was swimming, doing yoga, and a fitness class every week. Then I was put on bed rest and told to stop everything. An emergency cesarean, two months in the NICU, then bringing home a preemie threw all possibilities of exercise out the window. When I finally did return to a more vigorous workout routine, I was shocked. I was carrying more weight so I felt like my center of gravity was off and things I once could do were now a challenge. Start small. Go for a walk, breathe in the fresh air. Little by little, the weight comes off and you will feel more like yourself again. Little steps add up to big steps, but just remember to be kind to yourself.*

Regular exercise is an important part of self-care for several reasons. Regular exercise can:

- boost your mood and energy levels as "happy" hormones are produced;
- reduce stress and anxiety;
- promote a good night's sleep;
- reduce muscle tension and create feelings of relaxation;
- clear the mind and help you gain a better perspective to challenge depressing or anxious thoughts;
- increase self-confidence;
- give you a chance to meet others, have fun, and take some time for yourself;
- help you lose weight and tone your body.

ACTION PLAN: Activity Level

Try these strategies to increase your activity level:

- Talk to your doctor about any limitations on your activity.
- Choose an activity that works for you. You are more likely to be successful in sticking to an exercise plan if you do activities that you enjoy and that are practical.
- Be consistent. Shorter but regular exercise sessions are better than occasional long exercise sessions.
- Find childcare so that you can have some time to yourself while you exercise.
- Take your baby with you. Use a baby carrier, bike trailer, or stroller that lets you do your activities with your baby.
- Take a "mommy and baby" fitness class.
- Exercise with a friend or find out if there is a stroller-walking program in your community.
- Exercise at home. Take out exercise books or CDs from the library, look them up on YouTube, or use an app.
- Start with five minutes of activity—perhaps walking to the end of the block and back. If after five minutes you can keep going, then do that if you like, but it's not required. You only commit to those five minutes at first.

♥ *A front pack and a stroller are my new exercise equipment. A power walk in the morning works great. Baby just sleeps through it. And a stroller walk with my partner or my mom in the evening. We started off slowly because my hips really needed to tone up after being pregnant. Now we are rocking our walks at a quick pace. It'll be a great workout until my baby is big enough for me to get back to regular exercise.*

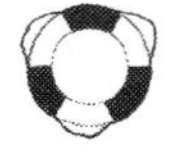

Sleep and rest

Sleep and rest are very important for both your physical and mental health. However, once you are home it can be difficult to get the sleep and rest that you need. Many women with preemies experience problems getting enough hours of uninterrupted sleep, in part because of the demands of caring for the baby. When you are sleep-deprived your mental health may suffer. It is worth the effort to work on getting more sleep and rest.

♥ *I was not one of those moms who sleeps when baby sleeps. We didn't have a big support system because my family lives halfway across the country. I had too much to do (pump, wash bottles, track milk volumes, make appointments) to take a nap. This backfired on me. I was running on roughly four hours of interrupted sleep in a twenty-four-hour period for weeks. I was sleep-deprived to the point where I felt like running away. I couldn't think straight, but I did not associate it with lack of sleep at the time. I thought I was going crazy. In retrospect, I know my feelings were totally linked to running on barely any sleep. I reached out to my husband and he started to take over some night feeds so I could sleep. Or he fed our daughter while I pumped so that we could both get sleep in between feeds. My distress went away after a few nights of decent sleep.*

ACTION PLAN: Sleep and Rest

Try these strategies to promote your sleep and rest:

- Ask for help. This may involve asking a friend or partner to mind the baby or take over some chores so that you can get to bed earlier or catch a nap. Many women have reported the difference that five hours of uninterrupted sleep can make to their anxiety, mood, and ability to cope.
- Create a bedtime ritual or routine. You may have to make some adjustments to your routine as the demands of your baby change. However, most of us settle down for sleep best when we have a routine that helps us to unwind and relax, such as taking a warm bath, light pleasure reading, listening to soft music, or doing breathing or relaxation exercises. Have a wind-down period before going to bed.

- Try to go to bed at a reasonable and consistent hour each night. This helps your brain and body to know when it should be feeling awake and when it should be feeling drowsy.
- Value your rest. Even if you don't fall asleep, lying down and resting is valuable.
- Remember that if you are getting up a lot during the night, you will need to take rest during the day to make up for lost sleep.
- Force yourself to lie down at least once during the day while your baby is sleeping. Even twenty minutes is helpful, forty-five minutes is refreshing, and ninety minutes would be the wonderful completion of a sleep cycle.
- Give yourself permission to sleep or rest. Manage daily stresses by making a to-do list for the next day, well in advance of bedtime. Give yourself permission to leave tasks until tomorrow.
- Adjust expectations of yourself. If you do not change your standards to reflect the changes that having a preemie baby makes in your life, it will be difficult to devote time to get the rest or sleep you need.
- Make where you sleep comfortable and relaxing. Most people sleep best in a dark, quiet, and somewhat cool bedroom. Napping on the lumpy couch might not be the most restful place.
- Reduce or cut out caffeine and do not have any within two hours of bedtime. Some experts recommend avoiding any caffeine after 4 p.m.
- If you exercise, stop at least two hours before bedtime. Although exercising regularly can help you to get deeper sleep, doing it too close to bedtime can make it more difficult to fall asleep because your body is still too revved up.
- Avoid being hungry or eating too heavily before bed. Consider a light carbohydrate snack, such as cereal, if you are hungry before bed.

♥ *My anxiety was at an all-time high when I was extremely sleep-deprived. I would notice that I was feeling extra anxious and I would think about it and, sure enough, I had had less sleep in days prior. I also learned not to place too much emphasis on my feelings during those times. I would ask my partner to remind me that I felt this way because I was tired and that I would feel better once I caught up on rest.*

My partner and I traded naps in the early days, which helped us both keep going. With our first daughter, I breastfed her, so I was the only one getting up. However, with our preemie, I was exclusively pumping so my partner and I shared the responsibility. I had some sad feelings about having to pump over breastfeeding our baby, but the sharing of the nighttime feedings was a silver lining. When I got up with our son, I could be very present and really soak him in, in the quiet of night, because I was a bit more rested.

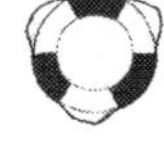

Time for you and your partner

An area most likely to be neglected after you become a parent is taking time for yourself. This may be especially true if you have a preemie. For some women, learning to take time for themselves can be a difficult habit to develop and can even cause feelings of guilt. Men often juggle working and providing for the family while trying to support their spouse and look after themselves. You might be a single parent. It can be challenging to take time for yourself when you have so many things that need to be done. However, taking time to care for yourself is an important part of self-care and a necessary part of mental wellness after discharge home.

ACTION PLAN: Relaxation

Try these strategies to take time for yourself and to relax:

- Do something for yourself that makes you feel good or joyful. Daily uplifts can protect people from the negative physical and mental effects of stress. Often when people feel stressed or pressed for time, they cut back on all of the pleasurable ingredients that make life enjoyable, but this is not helpful. No one does well if the only ingredients in their day or week are duties and chores.
- Find more time for yourself. Some women have been able to do this by adjusting their expectations, for example, doing certain chores less frequently or thoroughly. Consider dropping some non-essential tasks from your to-do list, for example, using a premade dish or prepackaged food for a meal. You could spend the saved time doing something for yourself. Control what you can and let go of what you can't.

- Ensure that you have periods of downtime or relaxation in your day. Make use of moments when your baby is content or asleep. Don't rush around without breaks or time to unwind from morning until bedtime. This may involve scaling back what you hope to accomplish in a day. Even slowing your pace and being more "in the moment" as you move through your daily activities can help. Here are many suggestions for break time:

  Apply scented lotion
  Browse in the library
  Color
  Contact an old friend
  Daydream
  Do a guided visualization
  Do a word puzzle
  Drink tea from a real teacup
  Eat a warm bowl of soup
  Enjoy a moment of silence
  Garden
  Go for a walk
  Keep a journal
  Knit
  Let someone hold you
  Listen to your favorite music
  Look at old photographs
  Meditate
  Paint your nails
  Paint or draw a picture
  Pet your cat or dog
  Practice progressive muscle relaxation
  Practice relaxed breathing
  Read
  Rest with a cozy blanket
  Rock in a rocking chair
  Sit in the sun
  Sit still and quietly for five minutes
  Sit in a place of worship
  Spend time in nature
  Take a bath
  Watch a movie
  Watch the sunset

- Ask for or accept help from others. Don't suffer in silence. Be open about your needs. It will benefit everyone in the long run.
- Connect with others. Spend time on relationships, whether writing a brief email, posting on Facebook, calling or meeting a friend for coffee, spending time with your partner, and so on.
- Have fun. Play can be spontaneous, give you a break from daily duties, and can involve others or be done on your own.
- Renew your relationship with your partner. You are stronger together. Find time to spend time alone together without baby. Reach out to your supports for babysitting. This is often difficult for preemie parents who are concerned others may not have the skills to care for their vulnerable little

one. Use people you trust and teach them the special ways to take care of your baby. Start with short breaks and gradually build. One word of caution for couples that are able to find time to reconnect sexually: Even if you are breastfeeding, you can get pregnant if you do not use birth control. So, unless you want another wee one in your family, use contraception. Getting pregnant too soon after having a premature baby can result in the next baby being more premature than the first baby. Your body needs to rest and heal before becoming pregnant again. Talk to your doctor about pregnancy spacing. Discuss using birth control pills with your doctor, as they can affect breast milk supply. If you are unsure which contraception to use, please see your doctor.

Working on time for yourself and your partner will boost your life preserver and help you stay afloat. Make it a priority!

♥ *My partner and I felt like ships passing in the night for many months after we brought our baby home from the hospital. We looked for small ways to reconnect and committed to them. We would sit on the couch together for at least fifteen minutes every day. I tried to tell him how much I appreciated how hard he was working to support our family and he did the same. Some of our talks were about being proactive and discussing what we would do if one of us started to feel really disconnected. Sometimes, it was refreshing to just watch our sleeping children and marvel at how amazing they are and how blessed we are to have them. We also talked about how far we had come from when we were in the NICU, which gave us a lot of valuable perspective.*

♥ *My husband and I always joke that we are rocking the parenting side of our relationship but slacking on the husband-wife side. We have birthday parties and swimming lessons to go to, whereas before our daughter was born, we had a wide-open schedule to do whatever we wanted. At the end of the day, we are exhausted and often don't have much left for each other. We weren't comfortable leaving the house at the beginning, so we planned "at-home date nights." We lit the fireplace, made dinner, sat on the carpet and talked. We've made the best of out of it but continue to have to prioritize "us time" amongst the busyness of parent life.*

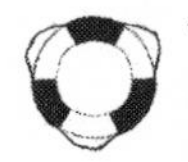

Support

Social support plays a very important role in helping people make it through the many life changes that go along with becoming a parent. This is even more true when you come home with a preemie. Healthy relationships are a protective factor against many mental health challenges. Increasing and strengthening healthy, supportive relationships is a strong strategy for well-being.

There are many forms of support, such as emotional, practical, and social. Chapter 1 addressed a variety of ways you can build your support systems. Here is a reminder of some of the suggestions:

Types of support

	Definition	Questions to ask yourself
Practical Support	The ways in which you get help with basic tasks and completing your to-do list. For example, assistance from family, responsible teenager next door, hired help.	Who can you call for help when you really need it? Who can help with errands, everyday household tasks, childcare, and so on?
Social Support	The groups or people you turn to for socialization and companionship. For example, immigrant women's society, NICU parents, and adult friends.	With which groups do you feel a sense of belonging and companionship? Which friend(s) could you reconnect with? What other moms or dads could you connect with?
Emotional Support	The people or groups you reach out to for emotional or spiritual support. For example your best friend, counselor, psychologist, religious leader.	Who in your life makes you feel good about yourself and reminds you of your strengths? Who can or do you talk to, especially about your worries and concerns?

There are several sources of these types of support you might consider:

- **Family:** partner, parents, siblings, extended family.
- **Friends:** friends, coworkers, other parents you met in the NICU.
- **Wider community:** neighbors, religious communities, community and recreational centers.

- **Support groups:** postpartum support groups, breastfeeding, young, or single moms groups, immigrant women's societies, cultural groups, aboriginal centers, social media (for example, Facebook support groups for parents of preemies, parent-to-parent NICU support).
- **Hired support:** nannies, housekeepers, babysitters, doulas, postpartum help businesses, respite support.
- **Health care:** health hotlines, family doctor, pediatrician, public health nurse, psychologist, psychiatrist, counselors, social worker.

ACTION PLAN: Support

Try these strategies to build your sources of support:

- Make a list of the people in your life who can provide support in each of the main areas. A table below provides space for you to list who can give you different types of support and also to write down specifically what they can do to support you.

Your supports

Support	Person, group, agency	How they might help
Practical Support	1. 2. 3.	
Social Support	1. 2. 3.	
Emotional Support	1. 2. 3.	

Perhaps you are hesitant to ask for the support that you need. You might think that other people should know what you need. Or you think that other people are too busy. Just ask! Be clear in what you need. What type of support do you seek? Hands-on help? Or just a friend to listen to you? Do you need one-time or weekly help? Put your needs on the table and ask. Many times, others don't understand the workload involved with parenting a preemie. With all the different kinds of supports available, someone will rise to your request and help you build your life preserver.

> ♥ *The friends we made in the NICU were some of our biggest supports because they just understood us in such a unique way. We are lifelong friends now and we feel so blessed that we gained a NICU family. We found that some family members had trouble understanding why it took us so long to get back on our feet after the NICU. However, we learned that people don't have to completely understand your situation to offer support. At first I was discouraged about some comments family members would make about things needing to get "back to normal." However, we were able to recognize that certain supports were good for certain things. So, we learned to use some of our supports for logistical things, some for childcare, getting organized, and so on. We leaned on some close friends, NICU friends, and professional supports to talk about challenges and emotional things.*

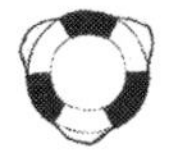

Spirituality

Spirituality is a basic human need. Spirituality connects us to something bigger than ourselves and helps us find meaning in life. It might include religious worship at a synagogue, temple, church, or mosque. You may reach out to your spiritual strengths through mindfulness, meditation, yoga, peaceful moments, private prayer, or time in nature. A spiritual person doesn't have to be religious.

Spiritual people have been found to be happier. They use their religion or belief system and values to understand the world and what is happening to them. They are able to see their situation and understand a reason for it. Finding meaning helps parents reframe their situation and challenges.

Why did this happen to me? God had a reason for giving me this special baby to love and nurture and help grow into a beautiful young man. We will coach him carefully and celebrate every success. God knew what I could handle.

ACTION PLAN: Spirituality

Try these strategies to support your spirituality:

- Follow your religious or cultural practices.
- Meditate, even for short periods. Use an app to guide you.
- Practice inhaling slowly and deeply through your nose and fully expanding your lungs. Hold your breath for a couple seconds and exhale through your mouth.
- Use the power of prayer.
- Read a spiritual book.
- Find a teacher or mentor to support your spiritual beliefs.
- Take up yoga.
- Reflect on your life and experiences through journaling.
- Walk outside and connect with nature.
- Pause to be in the moment and appreciate the beauty around you (for example, the smell of rain, the crunch of leaves under your feet, the beautiful view from a window).
- Practice thinking positively.
- Pause to reflect on the goodness in your life and be thankful.
- Look for strengths, not weaknesses.
- Demonstrate gratitude.

In a time when everything was so out of control, I found great comfort in believing that there was a higher power at play, taking care of our baby. These days, I'm so grateful for the experiences I had in the NICU because I feel like I have seen miracles take place. I feel like I have been changed as a mother, a partner, and a person.

When Your Life Preserver Isn't Enough

Mothers who have had a preterm birth experience have significantly higher levels of stress than women who deliver at term. They are at a higher risk for maternal mental health issues, such as anxiety and depression, and post-traumatic stress disorder (PTSD). Even fathers can experience these issues. This is due to the traumatic nature of a preterm birth, which can include actual or threatened serious injury or death to both the mother and the baby.

This section includes some of the common mental health issues and the symptoms you may experience. These mental health issues can affect mother-baby attachment and also your baby's development, so it is important to be able to recognize the symptoms in yourself or your partner, know what to do, and know how to get help. If you are not feeling like yourself, or if you notice your partner is not behaving as usual, reach out. Pay attention to your mental health. Ask your partner and friends if you seem like your usual self.

The good news is that help is available. Both women and men affected by mental health issues need not to suffer in silence. Treatment is available. With proper care and support you can fully recover.

Risk factors for mental health issues

You may be at greater risk of developing a mental health issue if you have:

- had a previous episode of mental illness such as anxiety, depression, bipolar, obsessive-compulsive disorder;
- a family member with a history of a perinatal mental illness;
- lack of support in caring for your baby, lack of sleep, exhaustion;
- marital or relationship stress;
- financial stress;
- health stress of your own, of a loved one, or of your baby;
- multiples, such as twins or triplets;
- type A or perfectionist personality.

Anxiety and worry

The many changes and uncertainties that parents experience following the birth of a premature baby contribute to some worry in almost all mothers and fathers. It's normal for parents to worry about their children. It's normal for parents of prematurely born children to experience stress while their baby is fragile and in the NICU.

> *Every hour in the NICU, I worried about my baby. Was he going to survive? Was he in pain? Was he gaining weight? As he got stronger, my worry never went away, but it did change. Now I worry about next week and the future. Will he be okay in school? Will he fall in love or get married? Worry never goes away. Welcome to parenthood.*

You went through a lot in the NICU. For many parents, the worry and anxiety doesn't end when they leave. You may experience fear of not being able to care for your baby at home. Your baby may have a setback or have to be rehospitalized or be given a new medical diagnosis. You are also undergoing changes in relationships, lifestyle, and may have financial worries and medical bills. Some parents worry more than others. Although some parents realize that their fears are exaggerated or unrealistic, it can be hard to stop thinking about them. At low levels, anxiety can be helpful for us—it can motivate us to work on tasks; it can increase our ability to focus, make us more alert, and help us avoid dangerous situations. However, when anxiety becomes intense, lasts for long, or interferes with our lives, seeking help is imperative. If excessive worry or fear is taking up a lot of time and energy and interfering with your quality of life, you likely have anxiety.

> *I was worried every minute of every day about my daughter's feeding. I counted every single milliliter that she drank and had a target amount recommended by our nurse that I prayed she would get to every day. She rarely got to that target amount and my worries grew. Many months later, when my daughter was eating solids and gaining weight like a champ, I still held those anxious feelings about her eating, and that target of 475 milliliters (2 cups) per day was burned in my memory. I sought help from a social worker who specialized in birth and pregnancy trauma and worked past those feelings with her support. Our journey as parents of preemies can be unpredictable and scary and is a steep learning curve. Reach out to your friends and family, and do not be ashamed to seek professional help.*

Symptoms of anxiety to monitor include:

- shortness of breath;
- chest pain or tightness;
- feeling as though your heart is pounding;
- lightheadedness;
- shaking;
- sweating or chills;
- nausea;
- numbness or tingling.

If your worry has progressed to include some of the symptoms above, it has likely developed into generalized anxiety. If these symptoms come on suddenly and are accompanied by an overwhelming sense of fear, it a panic attack. A panic attack is a "false alarm" of the body's stress-response system. If you think that your anxiety symptoms may be part of an anxiety disorder, talk to a health professional about the issue.

♥ *I gave birth four months ago to twenty-six-week-old twins. We spent more than ninety days in the NICU, with lots of ups and downs. After leaving the hospital I found it hard to find the time to care for myself. I wasn't getting much sleep as the babies were demanding and fed every three hours. I was feeling very uneasy and agitated at times. I felt breathless, my heart raced, I was sweaty and had tingling in my hands and feet. I thought I was having a heart attack and was going to die. The first time this happened I went to the emergency room, but I was sent home saying that my heart was just fine and that is was probably a panic attack.*

I became very fearful of having these episodes. They began to happen more and seemed to come from out of the blue. They mostly occurred when I left the house, and particularly in the supermarket or crowded places. I started to avoid leaving the house. I did not understand how this could be happening to me—I had always been so independent. I began having difficulty enjoying my babies.

I was scared to tell anyone about these thoughts and fears in case people thought I was crazy. Thank goodness my mother noticed something was really wrong. She convinced me to discuss it with my doctor, who helped me get the treatment I needed. Over the next couple of months, my symptoms decreased and I was able to enjoy being with my babies more and more.

Anxiety can be accompanied by depression. Part of the reason for this may be that it is depressing to be anxious all the time. The symptoms of depression can overlap with the symptoms of anxiety. Keep reading for more information on depression.

While everyone worries to some extent, the worry can become excessive and overwhelming for some people. Some women with excessive worry during pregnancy or following the birth have never before considered themselves to be worriers. Other women who have a history of worry find that their symptoms return or worsen.

In many cases, this excessive worry will also be associated with uncomfortable physical symptoms such as:

- restlessness, feeling "keyed up" or "on edge";
- fatigue;
- difficulty concentrating;
- irritability;
- muscle tension/aches/soreness;
- sleep problems.

Getting information or reassurance from other people provides only temporary relief, then the worry starts again or worry about something else begins. The excessive worry consumes a great deal of daily life and interferes with activities. Excessive worry seems to occur without triggers and is often based on thoughts of worst-case scenarios. These invasive thoughts will seem impossible to control.

Parents who find that they spend many of their waking hours worried and that it is difficult to "shut off" the worry may have excessive worry. These excessive worries and fears can snowball into anxiety, which may affect your behavior.

You may have excessive worry if:

- you are unable to leave the baby with others or out of your sight;
- you wake at night frequently to check if baby's still breathing;
- you are unable to sleep because of worry that something will happen to your baby while you are asleep;
- you call your doctor repeatedly;
- you repeatedly ask others for reassurance;
- you repeatedly search the internet for medical information because you worry excessively about your baby's health.

Unfortunately, these behaviors, while used with good intentions, ultimately serve to keep the anxiety going. It is important to remember that all of us experience anxiety from time to time, most typically when we feel threatened. Some experiences will trigger anxiety in most of us.

Seeking help for anxiety

Getting help is very important. Unfortunately, many people dealing with anxiety following the birth of a premature baby do not seek treatment. Some find it difficult to confide in their health care provider about their feelings. They may fear that they will be labeled or not taken seriously. Some may feel ashamed about not feeling happy like people expect them to be. Some fear others may think they are unable to care for their baby. Some have scary thoughts about harming the baby or find that their anxiety prevents them from attending appointments. Any of these can be a barrier to seeking help. It can be even more challenging for men, as they are less exposed to health care services that might identify problems and are often more reluctant to ask for help. Another barrier may be cost, as some professional services are expensive and not covered by insurance. Talk to your doctor about options you can afford.

ACTION PLAN: Anxiety

Try these strategies to address anxiety:

- Make small changes to improve self-care, as described in the beginning of this chapter. This is one of the most important steps you can take to start feeling better.
- Increase your circle of social support.
- Attend support groups.
- Get counseling.
- See your doctor for regular follow-up, and perhaps prescribed medication.

There are effective treatments available for excessive worry/anxiety following the birth of a premature baby. Telling your health care professional about your symptoms is the first step toward getting the help you need to feel better. For many, excessive and uncontrollable worry is part of a treatable anxiety disorder. Your health professional can help you to determine whether this applies to you. Speak to your health care provider about treatments options available.

♥

It is really important to understand how normal these feelings are. Anxiety is a huge barrier for parents worried that people will think they can't take care of their baby. Professionals view reaching out for help as a strength.

Looking back, I likely needed help with anxiety after the birth of my first child, but I was too scared to tell anyone because I didn't want anyone to think I couldn't take care of my baby. When my second child was in the NICU, I knew I was going to need some help with my anxiety. I openly talked with a psychologist and I put strategies in place. I felt vulnerable at first, but my psychologist assured me that what I was feeling was common and normal. It took a long time to get to a place where my anxiety was manageable, but doing so has changed my whole life and has helped me be a much more present parent.

Depression and postpartum depression

Up to 25 percent of women experience postpartum depression (PPD). Having a premature baby increases your risk. Although having a baby brings many positive things to one's life, it also requires a lot of adjustments to our priorities and how we see the world. The postpartum period creates major change in your life especially with sleep, routines, roles and relationships.

Depression following the birth of the baby affects a woman's mood, behavior, thoughts, and physical well-being. Signs and symptoms of depression are included in the following chart.

Symptoms of depression

Feelings associated with depression
• extreme sadness • irritability • anger • guilt • fear • worthlessness • hopelessness • overwhelmed • lack of joy in being with your baby • lack of joy in being a parent
Behaviors associated with depression
• inability to take pleasure in activities that you used to enjoy • inability to laugh at funny things • crying for no apparent reason • blaming yourself for things that are out of your control • experiencing low energy • having trouble concentrating • sleeping a lot more or less than usual • eating a lot more or less than usual • withdrawing from family, friends, and social contact • thinking of harming yourself, your baby, or others

! If you are you experiencing thoughts about harming yourself or someone else, seek help immediately.

Sometimes when people feel very anxious and/or depressed and hopeless, they have thoughts about harming themselves or others. If this is happening to you, it is very important that you tell someone you trust about these thoughts and make an urgent appointment to see your family doctor. Call your local mental health crisis hotline. If you are worried that you may be unsafe, please call 911 or go to the nearest emergency room.

! If you are seeing or hearing things, feel hopeless, have extremely confused thoughts, or feel like you can't trust anyone, call 911 or go to the nearest emergency room.

The above symptoms might indicate postpartum psychosis. These symptoms are very rare, but can occur after having a baby. If you are experiencing any of these symptoms, you need to get help immediately. Please call 911 or go to the nearest emergency.

Depression risk factors. Many women are surprised and disappointed when they find themselves feeling depressed following the birth of their baby. The trauma of experiencing a preterm birth can lead to maternal depressive symptoms. There are other challenges that can make depression more likely during this time.

These include:

- changes in relationships with partner, family, and friends;
- significant role changes in becoming a mother;
- career or work interruption;
- lifestyle changes, such as financial pressures;
- fatigue and sleep deprivation;
- caring for a new baby along with other responsibilities;
- significant physical changes to a woman's body such as weight gain, changes to the breasts;
- significant changes in hormone levels.

Women with a history of depression or anxiety are at higher risk for PPD. These women may have chosen or were directed to stop taking their medications prior to or during pregnancy. This may lead to an increase in anxiety or depressive symptoms after delivery.

Depression affects baby. Untreated PPD has been shown to affect the relationship between parents and their baby. Parents with depression feel disconnected from their baby and lack the normal joy of bonding. Parents with depression will smile less at their baby and will talk less to their baby. They may be insensitive or less responsive to their baby. These parental behaviors will impact your baby's development. The combination of parental depression and infant prematurity creates even more risk for less optimal infant outcomes.

♥

I didn't have the energy for my daughter. She was fed and dressed, but that was it. That's all the energy I had. We couldn't share happy times together. I felt worthless as a mother. My guilt made it worse. And then I'd feel more depressed and hopeless. It was like a vicious cycle. I told my public health nurse about how I was feeling. She did a postpartum depression screen and found I was definitely experiencing it.

When mothers are depressed, they are less likely to play with and stimulate their baby. In response, these babies have less secure attachment and less trust. Studies of babies of mothers with depression tend to have behavioral difficulties, sleep disturbances, and delayed cognitive, language, emotional, and motor development. Treatment of depression is important for you and your baby. When mothers with depression receive therapy and infant stimulation advice, their infants demonstrate positive interactions during play, improved feeding behaviors, clearer cues, and improved sleep patterns and development. Reach out for help—for your sake and for your baby.

Fathers and depression. Research has focused on mothers and PPD. We know much less about fathers. More recently it has been found that fathers too can experience stress and depression during the NICU stay and following discharge. Changes in relationships, lifestyle, financial worries, and the pressure of feeling unable to support a partner—a provider/protector anxiety—are all factors. The experience of witnessing a traumatic birth or illness in mothers or baby can be a trigger. Men may feel that as fathers and providers, they need to be strong, cope well, and be in control. This pressure can be overwhelming and can lead to symptoms of depression.

♥ *No one asked about my partner's mental health, at any point, during or after the NICU. It was only after I started to get some help that I realized he was dealing with a lot of guilt about having to leave me in the operating room to follow our baby to the NICU, even though we made this decision together. He was also having a lot of flashbacks from medical procedures he saw performed on our baby in the first moments of his life. He said he felt silly to admit that he was struggling at all. He said that everything "happened" to the baby and me, so he didn't feel like he had the right to have any needs around his mental health. I had to remind him that he had to deal with the worry of losing his partner and his baby while staying strong for our other child at home.*

♥ *My husband was our rock through the pregnancy, NICU stay, and returning home. It wasn't until months later, when I was feeling stronger and our daughter was thriving, that he admitted he was struggling with it all. He sought out a professional to talk to and benefited from having a third party to share his feelings with. He was finally able to open up about the fears, worries, and experiences from this journey.*

Fathers often do not receive the same attention from health care professionals as mothers do in relation to anxiety or depression screening. Men may not express their emotions to avoid feeling vulnerable, weak, or incapable. Suppressed emotions are taxing to mental health. The wrong approach, but sadly the common approach by men, is to ignore these feelings of anxiety or depression. The father's mental health is just as important as the mother's.

ACTION PLAN: Depression

Try these strategies to address depression:

- Tell your health care professional about your symptoms. This is the first step toward getting the help you need to feel better.
- Make small changes to improve self-care, as listed earlier in this chapter. Get good nutrition, rest, and exercise. These are powerful ways to boost your mental health.
- Avoid drugs or alcohol.
- Set small, achievable goals.
- Ask your doctor about taking vitamins and omega-3 supplements. Omega-3 may also be obtained by increasing your intake of foods with omega-3, such as fish.
- Communicate with your partner, close friends, or family about how you are doing. Have key support people check in with you weekly.
- Keep regular appointments with a health care professional.
- Seek counseling. Many counselors, psychiatrics, and psychologists specialize in depression. Techniques to help anxiety and depression include cognitive behavioral therapy and interpersonal therapy. Psychotherapy may be individual, couple, family, or group. Ask your doctor and others for recommendations. Find someone who you feel comfortable with. You could interview various therapists until you find a good fit.
- Talk to your doctor or psychiatrist about prescribed antidepressant medication. You may have to try different ones or take different doses until you find what works. See your doctor regularly for follow-up. Talk to your doctor before you stop taking these medications.
- Consider doing both counseling and medication, as they may be more effective in combination.

Before I started treatment, my partner would come home from work and I'd still be in my pajamas and would not have eaten much. He encouraged me to talk to our doctor, but I waited because I thought this would pass. Looking back, I should have sought help sooner. Therapy helped me look at my life differently and work on solutions. The meds helped me get my life back.

It is a good idea to speak to your health care provider to find out about the treatment options that are available to you. Share this information with your loved ones, who can help you to think through the advantages and disadvantages of each option and how these would fit your life. You may want to consider getting help at home from family or friends until you start feeling better. Remember that the goal of treatment is to reduce your symptoms and increase your overall well-being so that you can do the things that are important to you. People will take different paths to feeling better and in the end any decision about treatment is very personal.

Post-traumatic stress

Many parents describe a point in time after NICU discharge where they reach a fragile mental state. For weeks or months in the NICU, you've been running on adrenaline, fear, anxiety, and may feel mentally and physically exhausted. You dig deep and find even more energy to weather the trip home. And then you hit a wall.

You go from living your life between home and the hospital. Everything else gets put on hold so that you can be with your baby. You are in survival mode. Coming home is wonderful. You no longer have to rush off to the hospital every morning, eat cafeteria food, or any of those things. But it can be a shock to the system. The hustle and bustle that you've grown accustomed to suddenly stops, and sometimes in those quiet moments of reflection, it all hits you.

When you no longer need to run on adrenaline and the fear and anxiety start to subside, some raw emotions may come to the surface. You may suddenly start feeling very unlike your usual self. You might feel irritable, lethargic, jumpy, or experience sleep disturbances. Your family and friends might notice the change in you.

If this happens to you, listen to the messages from yourself or others. Don't ignore these symptoms. You've likely experienced trauma for weeks and months: a stressful pregnancy, early or traumatic delivery, premature or sick newborn, feeling helpless and maybe even hopeless at times. These experiences are emotionally exhausting.

Yes, you are so happy to have your baby at home and life is much less stressful than before. But, that doesn't stop your mind from exposing just how difficult this was for you. In many ways, this feeling is like post-traumatic stress disorder (PTSD), which is not limited to war veterans or people who have witnessed a violent crime. Parents can experience PTSD after a NICU experience. Symptoms might vary over time and be triggered by memories or events that recall the scary experience. Symptoms of PTSD may start within a month of the traumatic experience, but could also present months or years later.

Symptoms of PTSD include:

- recurrent intrusive memories, flashbacks, dreams/nightmares;
- avoidance of thinking or talking about the traumatic experience;
- feeling hopeless, numb, negative, depressed, guilty;
- withdrawing from activities and people;
- trouble sleeping and concentrating;
- self-destructive behavior.

♥ *After the twins came home I had these bouts of tearfulness. Then I started experiencing frightening nightmares and vivid flashbacks to moments in the NICU. I kept reliving the time we saw the baby next to ours being resuscitated. My heart would be racing. I had trouble sleeping, which was interfering with my work. I didn't realize what was happening. I was the man in the house and I had to be the rock for my wife. I looked up my symptoms online and learned about PTSD following preterm birth. It described exactly how I felt. I am so glad I finally realized I was ill and got some help.*

You've been through a major critical event. Reach out to family and friends to discuss your feelings. If your partner is experiencing these signs, support them to get professional help. Treatment is available to get you back to your normal self and enjoying life again. Seek community resources, such as your family doctor, who may refer you to a psychologist, counselor, or psychiatrist. Many maternity clinics offer mental health resources for up to a year postpartum. Journaling, mindfulness, and meditation techniques have also been shown to help. Refer to the action plan for depression described above.

Vulnerable child syndrome and hypervigilance

Preemies are vulnerable at the beginning of their lives. But even when a premature baby is growing and developing well, some parents remain overly cautious and protective. Considering what you have been through, it is natural to want to protect your baby from illness and injury. Some parents become hypervigilant and worry unnecessarily, such as by taking your baby to the doctor at the slightest concern, discouraging your child's desire to actively explore the world around them, avoiding contact with other people and kids to prevent illness, and limiting participation in activities to avoid possible dangers. This overprotectiveness can impede your baby's normal development. They may become insecure, shy, dependent, and lack self-esteem. Vulnerable child syndrome is not a result of your infant's prematurity but is related to your parenting style.

♥ *Thank goodness for that nurse who kept telling me that my baby was "normal" and to treat him so. I would still be coddling him if it wasn't for her advice to get him into tummy time, stimulate him, and let him play by himself on a playmat.*

Once things have settled for your child and they are growing and developing well, you should begin to treat them like any other child, not the vulnerable preemie they once were. If you are struggling with this, talk to other parents who have had a premature baby, or your baby's doctor or nurse.

Navigating your new normal

All families respond differently to the traumatic event of having a premature baby. The goal is to return to your normal level of functioning following this traumatic event. Finding your new normal takes time and will be unique to you and your family. Personal strengths, strong relationships, and prior experience with adversity may help you recover more quickly. Taking one day at a time and taking care of yourself and your family are keys to success.

Plan to take your first vacation as a family within the next year. Vacations don't need to be elaborate or expensive. Can you get away for a couple of days or a week? Can you visit friends or family? Even a day trip for a picnic within an hour's drive from home will build your confidence and happiness. Extra planning is needed if your baby has special health needs, such as oxygen, but vacations are still possible. Vacations with your baby will help you enjoy your new normal.

Parents able to adapt and grow after having a premature baby report that they have a renewed perspective on life. Eventually, despite the stressors and lost dreams, they see the positive or find meaning in their experience. They learn to master the challenges that have been given to them.

♥ *Be prepared to be blown away at how strong and amazing your baby is. You've seen them through their most vulnerable time and now you can watch them grow and develop before your eyes. Every day is something new, and before you know it, they are giggling, sitting, eating avocado, saying "mama" and "dada," and climbing up the stairs. You may have a deeper gratitude and sense of excitement when these milestones occur because of the road you've traveled.*

♥ *Yes, my daughter has cerebral palsy and needs splints and help to walk. But that is not her full story. She is brilliant and loves to read. She is funny and likes to tell jokes. She is very loving and has lots of friends. She just can't walk on her own. We are doing just fine. When life gave us lemons, we made lemonade.*

Families that reach a comfortable place in life with their premature baby might want to give back. This might include mentoring other parents, fundraising for the NICU, contributing to social media blogs, knitting hats for preemies, assembling care packages for new NICU parents, volunteering as a NICU cuddler, and participating in World Prematurity Day (November 17) or local events. These activities help parents find a new sense of purpose and fulfillment. When you share your story in a positive light, you help yourself and someone else see the possibilities.

Now it's my turn to give back. After a year at home, I was ready. I became an NICU peer mentor and volunteer a couple of times a month. It gives me great joy to help other families on their NICU journey.

Families that are able to bounce back after challenge or tragedy learn important life lessons and coping strategies. When faced with future challenges, these families tend to be more resilient and resourceful. Read the powerful, inspiring stories from the families who contributed to this book in chapter 8.

Final Thoughts

In the spaces below, note a few new strategies you will try to build your life preserver.

1. ______________________________

2. ______________________________

3. ______________________________

You made it through the NICU experience, only to go home and have to continue to be so careful. You wonder if you will ever have that experience that every parent wishes for with their newborn. Lack of sleep, follow-up doctor's appointments, pumping, and feedings take their toll. I was lucky that I had great support and strong spiritual beliefs to help me through this. I saw a great psychologist to help me reframe the NICU experience and boost my ability to cope with PTSD. Eventually the dust settled. Our daughter is now thirteen months old. I have been so filled with joy seeing her grow, surpass milestones, and blossom into a feisty, happy child. The good memories start to outweigh the bad and you look back and can't help but be grateful for the experience. Each day the sun rises and you are all one day stronger than you were the day before.

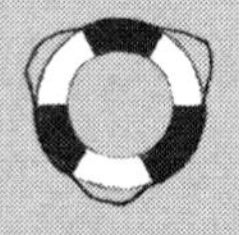

EXPERT TIPS

Here are the key strategies to navigate the journey

- Take good care of yourself so that you can take good care of your baby.
- Develop a support system.
- Speak openly about your feelings and what you need.
- Know the signs of excessive worry/anxiety, PPD, and PTSD.
- Monitor yourself and your partner for signs of anxiety and depression.
- Don't hesitate to seek professional help for mental health concerns.
- Start living your life with your baby.
- Find meaning in your experience.

8

NAVIGATING THE FIRST YEAR
Stories of Triumph

THE FIRST year of a preemie's life has its ups and downs, like a boat ride on rough or stormy seas. Premature babies are challenging to care for and need considerably more parent time and attention than full-term babies. Many premature babies have lingering health issues that take time to resolve. Setbacks and rehospitalizations are common. A simple cold can mean going back on oxygen. The health and development of premature babies requires close monitoring.

Taking home a premature baby can be a difficult transition. It takes a lot of patience and hard work for premature babies to recover, heal, and grow. Parenting a preemie can be hard work. Often parents must learn special care techniques to support their preemie's unique needs. Parents often turn to the internet for health information and answers to their questions. Exhaustion, worry, and uncertainty are common feelings. Parents need reliable information and support to stay healthy themselves.

We hope that that the proven effective and extensive recommendations in this book help smooth the turbulent waters of the first year with your baby. We hope that the strategies help you find the strength and confidence you needed to be the best parent you can be. We hope your baby is healthy, happy, and developing well. Best wishes as you and your baby start year two. You have done an amazing job to weather the first year. Remember to enjoy life together and have lots of fun.

In our work with families we noticed that parents love to hear from other parents. Parents felt relief knowing that they were not the only parents experiencing this preemie journey. The advice from other families was highly regarded and parents appreciated hearing others' expressions and descriptions of their experiences. This sharing helped families feel less alone. We knew that this preemie parent book would not be complete without their voices. We extend our heartfelt gratitude to our parent team for enriching this book with their lived experiences and advice. They willingly shared their feelings, pride, tears, tips, and encouragement. They did this to help other parents sail through the first year.

We end this book with their stories of survival and great accomplishment. You can literally feel their love and pride of what their once-premature baby has been through and become.

♥ **Alexandria** entered the world at thirty weeks' gestation and 1,100 grams. In the sixty-three days she spent in the NICU, she persevered through NEC and allergic colitis. Prior to discharge, I felt strongly that she suffered from reflux, so despite her doctor not recognizing the reflux, we implemented measures to ease her symptoms. Two days after coming home she suddenly went completely limp and blue while we were holding her upright after a feed. She had to be taken to hospital by ambulance and rehospitalized for two weeks. Finally, she got the official diagnosis of GERD, began medication, and started to get better.

We worried whether she would grow up to be "normal" or able to keep up with her peers. Some of our proudest moments have been watching her reach seemingly ordinary milestones—rolling over, her first steps, enjoying solids. Today, Lexi is a four-year-old preschooler, inquisitive, spunky, and every bit as saucy as she once was in the NICU. She loves dressing up as her favorite superheroes, being silly with her friends, extracting anything green from her dinner plate—all pretty normal four-year-old stuff. One of the greatest lessons of this NICU journey is that parents are their child's best advocates. Listen to your mommy or daddy instincts, those nagging voices or gut feelings are trying to tell you something.

DIANA

♥ **Emmett and Lucas**, my miracle babies, were born at twenty-five weeks and three days weighing 708 grams and 765 grams. Lucas was in the NICU for 132 days, though Emmett went home a little earlier. His stay was "typical," but Lucas was another matter—he was ventilated for seventy-two days, had

NEC, PDA [patent ductus arteriosis] surgery, and a brain hemorrhage. While we dealt with feeding and reflux and oxygen at home, it was on a milder scale. Once the boys were home and into the first year, their low muscle tone, especially in their shoulders, was a big challenge. They struggled with playing with their arms in the air and learning to hold their heads up took longer. Their strength was quite behind their peers. They are now in grade 2, looking and acting like typical seven-year-old boys. After all they had to overcome, they are thriving. They are the strongest, kindest, and funniest kids we know. Doctors told me that Lucas would never use the left side of his body; they said he would most likely have cerebral palsy and never run. But never underestimate the power of a preemie.

MICHELLE

Ethan was born at twenty-six-weeks' gestation weighing 640 grams. We spent 110 days in the NICU. Ethan was intubated for almost two weeks and on CPAP for a month and a half, had a PDA, brain bleed, and struggled with breastfeeding and bottle-feeding. Thankfully all these issues resolved themselves in the hospital. The biggest struggle we faced going home was adjusting to life outside the NICU. We measured every ounce of fluid he drank, weighed him every day, and found it difficult to put him to bed, as he no longer had monitors attached to him at all times. As the days and weeks went by, however, we became more comfortable and realized that the medical staff wouldn't have sent us home if they didn't believe he would succeed. Watching Ethan meet his milestones and become such a happy and healthy baby was wonderful. He is now two years old and a very active, adventurous, and curious toddler. Always trust your instincts and take things one day at a time. It does get easier.

LINDSAY AND MIKE

Jane was born at twenty-nine weeks after a long, scary battle with severe preeclampsia. She was 1,080 grams and spent fifty-nine days in two NICUs where she received care from some of the most talented and compassionate health care professionals. Feeding was our biggest challenge that didn't really sort itself out until she started solids. She wasn't able to breastfeed (despite five months of trying), so drank fortified breast milk. She gained weight very slowly and was not very efficient with her bottle. We tried everything and finally, around six months, with the support of an occupational therapist, she started to figure it out. Starting solids was a game changer for us. Jane is now almost two, as healthy as can be, and the most energetic, sassy, happy girl we know. She talks up a storm, loves the Canadian flag, peeing in the potty, jumping in puddles, and eating snacks. These little miracles are a special kind of magic. Give them time, they will find their way.

SARAH AND BRYAN

♥ **Leinah** was born at twenty-three weeks and one day, 500 grams and thirty centimeters long. She was in distress, breech, and coded a few minutes after the emergency C-section. We stayed 155 days in three different NICUs, where she faced uncountable health issues, including a bowel perforation and a massive pulmonary hemorrhage that required a second resuscitation. Defying all odds, Leinah came home on room air and exclusively mouth-fed. Today she is a smiley and feisty sixteen-month-old, a year corrected age, with few delays in speech and feeding. For sure the five first months were the most challenging. Dealing with the possibility of losing her, seeing her so small and already going through so much was heartbreaking, but every day is a highlight. Leinah has taught us that being alive is a gift. Just BELIEVE. Even when the game seems to be hard or already lost. Do not allow anyone to label your baby, trust your gut, take care of yourself, advocate and fight at your baby's side. No matter what, keeping believing. And know that although some journeys are shorter than others, each life is worth fighting for.

FLAVIA AND DANIEL

♥ **Kingston and Jackson** were born on Christmas Day at exactly twenty-nine weeks, weighing 1,020 and 1,162 grams, respectively. Our story actually started early on in our pregnancy with the diagnosis of twin transfusion syndrome. After multiple trips between two major cities we had in-utero surgery to save our twins' lives. After their birth, we weren't able to hold our boys for nine long days. During their NICU stay, they were ventilated on oxygen for seventy-three days, at times in isolation, had hernia surgery, eye problems, heart complications, rotation between multiple hospitals, and terrible reflux and feeding issues. Our health care provider wouldn't cover our twins given their state of health at the time of our application (at forty-five days old). We urge parents to set up medical within the first thirty days of their child's life. After 113 days in the NICU, our twins were discharged with chronic lung disease, follow-ups with cardiology, reflux and feeding issues, and with a whopping prescription bill of $600-plus monthly. An amazing transition team helped us through the next months at home. Our boys are now almost two years old. They are incredibly resilient, tough, and the happiest little guys you've ever seen. We are blessed.

HEATHER AND JASON

Mama was born at over twenty-seven weeks, she was 905 grams, tiny but with a huge fighting spirit. She stayed a total of eighty-nine days in two different hospitals. She did well in the NICU, but had a flu that kept her an extra two weeks. Taking her home and not relying on the monitors to help keep her safe was scary, but thank God it worked out well. Our greatest joy was seeing Mama excel at each stage of her life, meeting the milestones with no stress, but at her own time. She's now two years old, and most days I forget the journey because of how well she's turned out. Enjoy each day no matter how bleak or scared you feel, as there is always a light at the end of that tunnel.

ANNY AND MICHAEL

Noah was born at twenty-seven weeks, weighing 800 grams. This came as a shock because our first child was born full-term. Noah spent sixty-six days in two NICUs and faced challenges such as breathing issues, ROP, PDA, feeding issues, reflux, and a hernia repair. He is now an amazing two-year-old with the same strong, fighting spirit we were always so inspired by and he is developmentally on par. It was hard to balance the needs of our older child and believing that Noah was actually okay. But we know that we gained more than we lost through our NICU journey and it changed who we are as people, as parents, and as a family. We are grateful every single day. We believe that NICU parents are among the strongest and most resilient there are. Congratulations on your miracle. You got this.

NICOLE AND MICHAEL

Wally was our first baby, born at twenty-six weeks' gestation, weighing 766 grams. His early arrival was a big surprise and we'll never know for sure what caused it. We spent 113 days in three NICUs. He developed many of the typical medical concerns of a micro-preemie, such as retinopathy of prematurity, necrotizing enterocolitis, suboptimal growth, feeding issues, GERD, and several lung, breathing, and related sleep issues. When we felt overwhelmed, it helped us to step back and try to remember that every difficult moment would pass. He was on and off breathing supports for almost two years. However, he was a very feisty baby and did not let his early experiences prevent him from growing into a happy, healthy, now four-year-old boy. Finally being able to take him out, to experience things together as a family, felt terrific.

AMANDA

♥ **William and Alexander** were born at twenty-six weeks by emergency C-section with Alexander weighing 992 grams, and William weighing 682 grams. William had to be reintubated several times and had severe ROP that was treated with injections. He then had laser eye surgery, and severe reflux that caused oral aversion. Alex had intestinal issues that affected his breathing. Alex came home after four months in the NICU, and William spent an additional two weeks at the Children's Hospital following a surgery. William came home on oxygen and with a feeding tube, which made home life complicated. Our biggest success was helping William wean from his feeding tube. They are now ten months old corrected age and love crawling around and stealing one another's toys. Having a preemie is a challenge, but also an unexpected gift. The first time we were woken up by a crying baby at night I was filled with wonder and gratitude that our babies were home.

CANDACE AND IAN

ACKNOWLEDGMENTS

WE ACKNOWLEDGE the selfless dedication and contributions of our neonatal parent team. These parents helped us set the book priorities through focus groups, provided passionate and powerful stories, and reviewed chapters for relevance and completeness. With their lived experiences, these parents helped the book's content come alive.

We would like to acknowledge our own families for their support, encouragement, and patience as we tackled this monumental project. Many times, book-writing took precedence over family meals, household duties, and grocery shopping. No one complained, not even our dogs! We were always in the company of our fur babies, Kipper, Guinness, and Stella, who provided pet therapy, distraction, and much-needed breaks.

We thank our reviewers for their time to reflect on our work and provide editorial comments. We also want to thank our illustrator Kaylie Sauverwald, who took on this project while wrapping up the final year in her visual communications design degree. Her artistic talent with babies was a delight to discover. We hope this project catapults her career!

As novice book writers, we are incredibly grateful for the expertise of Page Two Strategies, our publishing consultants. Having previously published mostly academic work, writing for a parent population was a new challenge. Page Two helped us find our expert voice in parent-friendly language. They demystified the publishing process and were extremely easy to work with. Without their critical eye to details and timelines, this book would have been much longer and never completed!

Tammy would also like to acknowledge Mount Royal University for granting her a year sabbatical to move this project from a vision to reality.

We'd like to acknowledge a kind stranger we met on our first writing retreat. Taken in by our enthusiasm and vision, he provided us with a good bottle of red wine to sip by the fireplace as we conceptualized the beginnings of this book. Thoughts flowed very freely...

We also express our gratitude to one another. Our educational, career, and personal paths have intersected multiple times. We've completed two degrees at the same two universities; we've worked on the same team; we've each been in a managerial position over the other; we both had two children; and we both have a love for golden retrievers. We were destined to work together on a project of this magnitude. Coauthoring can have its challenges, but we managed to write, edit, debate over what's in and what's out, and we're still close friends and colleagues. No one else would have put up with our verbose writing style, perpetual interruptions, out-of-the-box thinking, and domineering passion about preemies and parents.

INDEX

Note: P *indicates Picture/Illustration and* T *indicates Table*

ABOUT THE AUTHORS

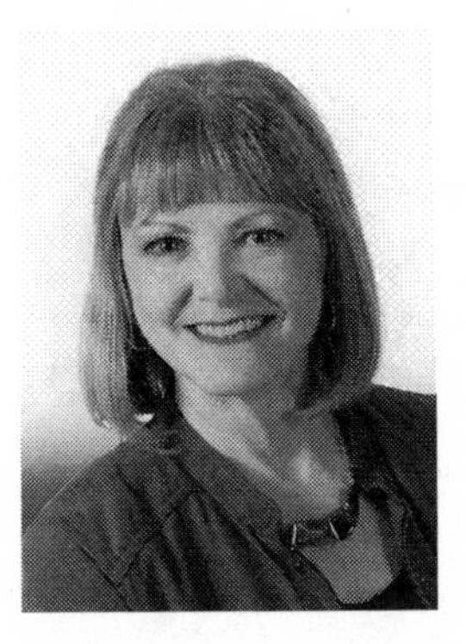

KAREN LASBY'S more than thirty-five-year nursing career includes NICU roles as bedside nurse, transport nurse and educator, pediatrics, pediatric intensive care, and community health. Karen leads a specialized nursing team in post-discharge follow-up of extremely premature infants and their families, the only team of its kind in Canada. She has presented locally, nationally, and internationally on the topics of premature babies, neonatal oral feeding, and NICU-to-home transition. She has been the co-investigator in several research studies examining outcomes for very low birth weight infants and has published several professional articles on maternal work in the NICU, neonatal transition, and gastroesophageal reflux. An educator for nearly thirty years, Karen has taught, written instructional material, and produced online courses for neonatal nursing programs. Formerly the president of the Canadian Association of Neonatal Nurses, she served on this national board for twelve years, and on the board of the Council of International Neonatal Nurses for three years. Karen has a master's degree in nursing and a neonatal nursing specialty certification with the Canadian Nurses Association and her work has been recognized by the Canadian Institute of Child Health and College & Association of Registered Nurses of Alberta.

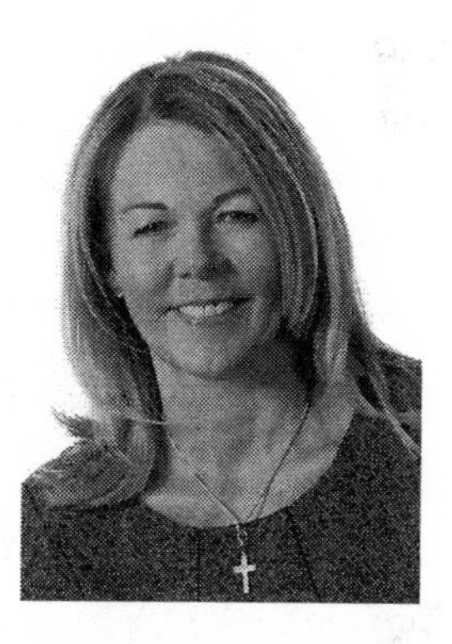

TAMMY SHERROW has a bachelor of science degree and a master's degree in nursing. During her thirty-three years as a nurse, the majority of her clinical experience has focused on the premature population, both in the NICU and in the community, as a staff nurse, educator, manager, and researcher. Tammy spent five years working with a specialized neonatal team following very low birth weight preemies and their families at home and knows firsthand the challenges they can face, especially during that first year. Tammy has published professional articles on the topics of parenting a preemie and gastroesophageal reflux management and has been a co-investigator in neonatal research projects on oral feeding and post-discharge outcomes. She has presented locally, nationally, and internationally on the topics of premature babies and NICU-to-home transition. She is an associate professor at the School of Nursing & Midwifery at Mount Royal University in Calgary, Alberta.

43174834R00192

Made in the USA
San Bernardino, CA
12 July 2019